Endocrine Pathology

Editor

PETER M. SADOW

SURGICAL PATHOLOGY CLINICS

www.surgpath.theclinics.com

Consulting Editor
JOHN R. GOLDBLUM

December 2014 • Volume 7 • Number 4

ELSEVIER

1600 John F. Kennedy Boulevard • Suite 1800 • Philadelphia, Pennsylvania, 19103-2899

http://www.theclinics.com

SURGICAL PATHOLOGY CLINICS Volume 7, Number 4
December 2014 ISSN 1875-9181, ISBN-13: 978-0-323-32684-1

Editor: Joanne Husovski
Developmental Editor: Donald Mumford

Surgical Pathology Clinics (ISSN 1875-9181) is published quarterly by Elsevier Inc., 360 Park Avenue South, New York, NY 10010. Months of issue are March, June, September, and December. Business and Editorial Office: Elsevier Inc., 1600 John F. Kennedy Blvd., Ste. 1800, Philadelphia, PA 19103-2899. Accounting and Circulation Offices: Elsevier Inc., 3251 Riverport Lane, Maryland Heights, MO 63043. Periodicals postage paid at New York, NY and at additional mailing offices. Subscription prices are $200.00 per year (US individuals), $233.00 per year (US institutions), $100.00 per year (US students/residents), $250.00 per year (Canadian individuals), $266.00 per year (Canadian Institutions), $250.00 per year (foreign individuals), $266.00 per year (foreign institutions), and $120.00 per year (international & Canadian students/residents). Foreign air speed delivery is included in all *Clinics*' subscription prices. All prices are subject to change without notice. **POSTMASTER:** Send address changes to *Surgical Pathology Clinics*, Elsevier, 3251 Riverport Lane, Maryland Heights, MO 63043. Customer Service: 1-800-654-2452 (US). From outside the United States, call 1-314-447-8871. Fax: 1-314-447-8029. E-mail: JournalsCustomerServiceusa@elsevier.com (for print support) and JournalsOnlineSupport-usa@elsevier.com (for online support).

Reprints. For copies of 100 or more, of articles in this publication, please contact the Commercial Reprints Department, Elsevier Inc., 360 Park Avenue South, New York, NY 10010-1710. Tel. 212-633-3874; Fax: 212-633-3820; E-mail: reprints@elsevier.com.

Contributors

CONSULTING EDITOR

JOHN R. GOLDBLUM, MD
Chairman, Professor of Pathology, Department
of Anatomic Pathology, Cleveland Clinic
Lerner College of Medicine, Cleveland Clinic,
Cleveland, Ohio

EDITOR

PETER M. SADOW, MD, PhD
Associate Director for Anatomic Pathology,
Pathology Residency Training Program;
Associate Director, Head and Neck Pathology,
Endocrine and Genitourinary Pathology;
Assistant Professor of Pathology, Pathology
Service, Massachusetts General Hospital,
Harvard Medical School, Boston,
Massachusetts

AUTHORS

ZUBAIR N. BALOCH, MD, PhD
Professor, Department of Pathology and
Laboratory Medicine, Perelman School of
Medicine, University of Pennsylvania,
Philadelphia, Pennsylvania

JUSTINE A. BARLETTA, MD
Assistant Professor, Department of Pathology,
Brigham and Women's Hospital, Harvard
Medical School, Boston, Massachusetts

GUIDO FADDA, MD, MIAC
Assistant Professor of Pathology; Head,
Cytopathology Section, Division of Anatomic
Pathology and Histology, Agostino Gemelli
School of Medicine and Hospital, Catholic
University, Rome, Italy

WILLIAM C. FAQUIN, MD, PhD
Department of Pathology, Massachusetts
General Hospital; Harvard Medical School,
Boston, Massachusetts

THOMAS J. GIORDANO, MD, PhD
Departments of Pathology and Internal
Medicine, and Comprehension Cancer Center,
University of Michigan Health System,
Ann Arbor, Michigan

NICOLE M. HARTFORD, CT(ASCP)
Pathology Service, Massachusetts General
Hospital, Boston, Massachusetts

VIRGINIA A. LiVOLSI, MD
Professor, Department of Pathology and
Laboratory Medicine, Perelman School of
Medicine, University of Pennsylvania,
Philadelphia, Pennsylvania

RICARDO VINCENT LLOYD, MD, PhD
Department of Surgical Pathology, University
of Wisconsin Hospital and Clinics, Madison,
Wisconsin

KATHLEEN T. MONTONE, MD
Professor, Department of Pathology and
Laboratory Medicine, Perelman School of
Medicine, University of Pennsylvania,
Philadelphia, Pennsylvania

ISOBEL C. MOUAT
Department of Pathology, University of
Michigan Health System, Ann Arbor, Michigan

VANIA NOSÉ, MD, PhD
Pathology Service, Massachusetts General
Hospital; Department of Pathology, Harvard
Medical School, Boston, Massachusetts

MARC P. PUSZTASZERI, MD
Department of Pathology, Geneva University
Hospital, Geneva, Switzerland

THEREASA A. RICH, MS
Clinical Cancer Genetics Program, The
University of Texas MD Anderson Cancer
Center, Houston, Texas

J.N. ROSENBAUM, MD
Department of Surgical Pathology, University
of Wisconsin Hospital and Clinics, Madison,
Wisconsin

ESTHER DIANA ROSSI, MD, MIAC, PhD
Attending Pathologist, Division of Anatomic
Pathology and Histology, Agostino Gemelli
School of Medicine and Hospital, Catholic
University, Rome, Italy

PETER M. SADOW, MD, PhD
Associate Director for Anatomic Pathology,
Pathology Residency Training Program;
Associate Director, Head and Neck Pathology,
Endocrine and Genitourinary Pathology;
Assistant Professor of Pathology, Pathology
Service, Massachusetts General Hospital,
Harvard Medical School, Boston,
Massachusetts

NAMRATA SETIA, MD
Surgical Pathology Fellow, Department of
Pathology, Brigham and Women's Hospital,
Harvard Medical School, Boston,
Massachusetts

MICHELLE D. WILLIAMS, MD
Associate Professor, Department of Pathology,
The University of Texas MD Anderson Cancer
Center, Houston, Texas

Contents

Poorly differentiated thyroid carcinoma (PDTC) has been recognized for the past 30 years as an entity showing intermediate differentiation and clinical behavior between well-differentiated thyroid carcinomas (ie, papillary thyroid carcinoma and follicular thyroid carcinoma) and anaplastic thyroid carcinoma; however, there has been considerable controversy around the definition of PDTC. In this review, the evolution in the definition of PDTC, current diagnostic criteria, differential diagnoses, potentially helpful immunohistochemical studies, and molecular alterations are discussed with the aim of highlighting where the diagnosis of PDTC currently stands.

Recent insight into the molecular mechanisms of thyroid carcinogenesis has led to studies involving newly directed antibodies. With the introduction of new molecular targeted therapies, these antibodies may represent useful predictors of therapeutic response in tumors unresponsive to radioiodine or insensitive to conventional antitumor therapies. These markers complement the development of markers that are able to discern benign from malignant entities, including hyalinizing trabecular tumors, oncocytic neoplasms, and follicular variant of papillary thyroid carcinoma. The use of antibodies directed to proteins generated by mutated genes may represent a cost-effective method for diagnosing and managing patients affected by thyroid tumors.

The complex interactions between immune cells and tumor cells in cancer play a major role in tumor development and subsequent patient outcomes. Different types of tumor-associated inflammatory cells (TAICs), such as dendritic cells, macrophages, lymphocytes, and mast cells, have been recognized for many years in several tumors; however, the role of TAICs in cancer is still not completely understood. This review article focuses on the major types of TAICs, including their general role in cancer and, more specifically, their role and distribution in thyrocyte-derived carcinomas.

This review focuses on the pathologic entities associated with hyperparathyroidism in humans. A discussion of the lesions, their embryology, and pathologic features is included. Immunohistology, cytopathology, and a brief overview of molecular aspects of the lesion are included.

Isobel C. Mouat and Thomas J. Giordano

Pathologists are highly skilled at the evaluation of adrenal neoplasms. Occasional adrenocortical tumors can be diagnostically challenging and supplementary tools can assist in these cases. Histologic and molecular studies support a model that includes 2 broad classes of adrenocortical carcinoma with distinct somatic genetic alterations and clinical outcomes. Pathologists should endeavor to grade adrenocortical carcinomas to assign each case into one of these 2 classes. Mitotic grading by mitotic counting and Ki-67 immunohistochemistry represent the most practicable and informative methods currently available.

Michelle D. Williams and Thereasa A. Rich

Seventy percent of parasympathetic paragangliomas arise in the head and neck and are nonsecretory. Awareness of the differential diagnosis based on location, overlapping morphology, and immunohistochemical profiles aids in the correct diagnosis, particularly on limited tissue samples. Moreover, 30% to 40% of head and neck paragangliomas are known to be associated with hereditary syndromes, with the succinate dehydrogenase enzyme family comprising the most frequent association. The pathologist's role is becoming increasing critical for facilitating optimal patient care beyond the initial tissue diagnosis of paraganglioma to include screening and documenting potential hereditary tumors requiring further patient counseling and testing.

J.N. Rosenbaum and Ricardo Vincent Lloyd

Pancreatic neuroendocrine neoplasms (Pan-NENs) are rare but clinically important lesions. Pan-NENs are known for and often categorized by their capacity to produce clinical syndromes mediated by the production of hormones. Despite sometimes presenting dramatically from excessive hormone production, not all Pan-NENs produce functional hormone, and they can pose diagnostic challenges to practicing pathologists. Distinguishing Pan-NENs from mimics can be crucial, because Pan-NENs carry different prognoses and have unique treatments available due to their specific biological properties. This article reviews the current categorization and features of Pan-NENs.

Peter M. Sadow, Nicole M. Hartford, and Vania Nosé

Endocrine tumors may present as sporadic events or as part of familial endocrine syndromes. Familial endocrine syndromes (or inherited tumor/neoplasm syndromes) are characterized by multiple tumors in multiple organs. Some morphologic findings in endocrine tumor histopathology may prompt the possibility of familial endocrine syndromes, and these recognized histologic features may lead to further molecular genetic evaluation of the patient and family members. Subsequent evaluation for these syndromes in asymptomatic patients and family members may then be performed by genetic screening.

SURGICAL PATHOLOGY CLINICS

FORTHCOMING ISSUES

Neuropathology
Tarik Tihan, *Editor*

Pathology Informatics
Anil Parwani, *Editor*

Genitourinary Pathology
Michelle Hirsch, *Editor*

Soft Tissue Pathology
Leona A. Doyle and Karen Fritchie, *Editors*

RECENT ISSUES

Pathology of the Medical Kidney
Anthony Chang, *Editor*

Cutaneous Lymphomas
Antonio Subtil, *Editor*

Cytopathology
Tarik ElSheikh, *Editor*

Hematopoietic Neoplasms: Controversies in Diagnosis and Classification
Tracy George and Daniel Arber, *Editors*

RELATED INTEREST

Otolaryngologic Clinics of North America
August 2014; Volume 47, Issue 4
Thyroid Cancer: Current Diagnosis, Management, and Prognostication
Robert L. Witt, *Editor*

NOW AVAILABLE FOR YOUR iPhone and iPad

Preface

Endocrine Pathology: Treading Water in a Shark Tank of Uncertain Malignant Potential

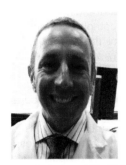

Peter M. Sadow, MD, PhD
Editor

A wonderful thing about endocrine-related diseases is that most of them make sense. Unlike the complicated molalities of the Loop of Henle or the mapping of the complex and vaguely specific geography of the brain, we can logically contemplate the mechanism of action of central to end-organ feedback of hormone regulation. If the body physiologically requires more calcium, calcium sensors tell the parathyroid to facilitate increased calcium absorption and secretion. To maintain homeostasis in body temperature and metabolism, thyrotropin-releasing hormone does a well-rehearsed dance with thyroid-stimulating hormone (TSH; or thyrotropin), which, in turn, greets the transmembrane TSH receptor in the thyroid to facilitate iodine uptake via the sodium iodide symporter and the production of thyroid hormone by thyrocytes. From thyroglobulin stores within thyroid follicles, there is secretion of thyroid hormone in its active form of triiodo-L-thyronine as well as in its primary form of thyroxine to be activated by cells in the body's periphery, resulting in intracellular modification of gene and protein expression via complexes associated with thyroid hormone receptor isoforms, and subsequently feeding back centrally to cool down additional secretion in times of plenty. For as much as we understand about endocrine physiology, a great deal is left to be discovered about endocrine pathophysiology, much of which centers around endocrine neoplasia.

Endocrine neoplasia comes in two main forms: lesions that are hormone-secreting and those that are nonsecreting. After that generalization, most other points remain rudimentary in our knowledge, especially in regard to the determination of biological behavior of these neoplasms, from incidental to low biological potential to potentially aggressive to frankly malignant.

Immunohistochemistry and more recently available molecular diagnostic tools have added layers to our documentation and understanding of gene expression profiles of endocrine neoplasms; however, for the most part, while helping us to more distinctly classify some tumor types, predicting behavior or response to particular treatment modalities is still, in many cases, elusive.

In this issue of *Surgical Pathology Clinics* devoted to Endocrine Pathology, we explore some emerging topics in this kinetic field as authored by several of its leaders accompanied by some rising stars. The breadth of topics includes the thyroid gland, revisiting the utility of immunohistochemistry in the diagnosis of malignancy, in addition to a thoughtful overview of the recently refined diagnosis of poorly differentiated thyroid carcinoma. Our discussion of the thyroid is rounded out by a foray into the role of the immune

Surgical Pathology 7 (2014) ix–x
http://dx.doi.org/10.1016/j.path.2014.09.001

surgpath.theclinics.com

system in the regulation of thyroid malignancy. Additional lightning rods for discussion are papillary thyroid carcinomas with high-grade features and the ever-troublesome follicular variant of papillary thyroid carcinoma. As additional molecular and outcomes data emerge from these entities, increasing in frequency of diagnosis, we can then make a more compelling story as to how to best classify them.

Accompanying the thyroid articles, authors explore our current understanding of parathyroid disease, pancreatic neoplasia, adrenal cortical disease, and paragangliomas, with particular attention to practical and molecular diagnostic approaches toward these organs that produce lesions of both certain and uncertain biological potential, with modulation of treatment and follow-up depending on the tumor morphology and molecular characterization.

Finally, we give an account of a diverse group of diseases under the auspices of familial endocrine syndromes. This group of neoplasias, having at least one major component of the syndrome as an endocrine-related malady, consists of some well-known entities with long-standing cause in addition to more recently described cohorts pending more thorough characterization. Included in the description of these syndromes are hallmark features and clues for the pathologist that may aid in the diagnosis of a specific syndromic entity as well as the basis to guide our clinical

colleagues toward broader exploration for associated abnormalities.

Although this issue is not exhaustive in its scope, it is my hope that the reader finds these topics to be both practical and informative. I am exceptionally thankful to the authors of these articles, who, along with their colleagues and trainees, have produced a truly thoughtful state of the field, and who make me very thankful and honored to be a member of the endocrine pathology community. I am particularly thankful for those authors who submitted their articles early and to those same authors who were patient as others submitted their articles a touch later. I am also very thankful to Joanne Husovski, who pretended not to be annoyed when I would reply to an e-mail four months later as if she had just sent the message. I am most thankful for many of my mentors in the field, especially Dr Vânia Nosé, who have participated in this undertaking, and I look forward to many more productive, collaborative years ahead.

Peter M. Sadow, MD, PhD
Pathology Service
Massachusetts General Hospital
Department of Pathology Harvard Medical School
55 Fruit Street
Boston, MA 02114, USA

E-mail address:
psadow@mgh.harvard.edu

Poorly Differentiated Thyroid Carcinoma

Namrata Setia, MD, Justine A. Barletta, MD*

KEYWORDS

- Thyroid • Carcinoma • Poorly differentiated • Insular

ABSTRACT

Poorly differentiated thyroid carcinoma (PDTC) has been recognized for the past 30 years as an entity showing intermediate differentiation and clinical behavior between well-differentiated thyroid carcinomas (ie, papillary thyroid carcinoma and follicular thyroid carcinoma) and anaplastic thyroid carcinoma; however, there has been considerable controversy around the definition of PDTC. In this review, the evolution in the definition of PDTC, current diagnostic criteria, differential diagnoses, potentially helpful immunohistochemical studies, and molecular alterations are discussed with the aim of highlighting where the diagnosis of PDTC currently stands.

> **Key Histologic Features**
> OF POORLY DIFFERENTIATED THYROID CARCINOMA
>
> - Areas of solid/trabecular/insular growth
> - Lack of nuclear features of papillary thyroid carcinoma in the poorly differentiated component
> - Convoluted nuclei
> - Increased mitotic activity (greater than or equal to 3 mitoses per 10 high power fields)
> - Coagulative tumor necrosis

OVERVIEW

Poorly differentiated thyroid carcinoma (PDTC) is a rare follicular cell–derived thyroid tumor accounting for approximately 0.5% to 7% of thyroid malignancies,[1,2] with the higher end of this range seen in iodine-deficient areas, such as Northern Italy. The average patient age is 55 to 70 years, and there is a slight female predominance (approximately 1.3–2.0 to 1).[1,3–5] The prognosis is significantly worse than that of papillary thyroid carcinoma (PTC) and follicular thyroid carcinoma (FTC).[1,3–6] Distant metastases are common,[1,3,6] with lung and bone the most frequent sites.[7,8] Because PDTC has been variously defined, the prognosis has not been entirely established; however, the 5- and 10-year survival rates of patients with PDTC as defined by the Turin criteria (discussed later) are approximately 70% and 50%, respectively.[1]

Histologically, PDTCs are invasive tumors that demonstrate areas of solid/trabecular/insular growth, a lack of nuclear features of PTC in these areas, and increased mitotic activity and/or necrosis.[5] Although immunohistochemistry may be used in the evaluation of cases in which a diagnosis of PDTC is considered, it is not required because the diagnosis of PDTC rests on histologic features.

EVOLUTION IN THE DEFINITION OF POORLY DIFFERENTIATED THYROID CARCINOMA

The term *poorly differentiated thyroid carcinoma*, was loosely used in older literature to describe undifferentiated thyroid carcinoma.[9] The diagnosis of PDTC as it is now known, however, was initially put forth in 2 seminal articles published in the early 1980s. At that time, follicular cell–derived thyroid carcinomas were considered histologically and prognostically as either well-differentiated (ie, PTC

The authors have no conflicts of interest to disclose.
Department of Pathology, Brigham and Women's Hospital, Harvard Medical School, 75 Francis Street, Boston, MA 02115, USA
* Corresponding author.
E-mail address: jbarletta@partners.org

Surgical Pathology 7 (2014) 475–489
http://dx.doi.org/10.1016/j.path.2014.08.001
1875-9181/14/$ – see front matter Published by Elsevier Inc.

or FTC) or undifferentiated/anaplastic thyroid carcinoma (ATC).[10] In 1983, Sakamoto and colleagues[11] identified a subset of thyroid carcinomas using architecture alone that had a poor clinical outcome in the absence of transformation to ATC. Histologically, these tumors were defined as having a nonglandular component as demonstrated by a solid, trabecular, or scirrhous (single cells or cords of cells within a fibrous stroma) architecture. Clinically, they demonstrated a behavior that was situated between that of indolent well-differentiated tumors and rapidly fatal ATC. The following year, Carcangiu and colleagues[12] described a histologic subset of thyroid carcinomas with a similar prognosis as described by Sakamoto and colleagues (ie, intermediate between well-differentiated carcinomas and ATC) that they referred to as poorly differentiated, or insular, thyroid carcinoma. Insular referred to the nests of tumor cells that were sharply demarcated from the adjacent stroma secondary to artifactual clefting, imparting an appearance similar to that of carcinoid tumors with an insular growth pattern. Although architecture was also a key component of the tumors in their cohort, in addition they described unique cytologic features (uniform small cells with a small amount of cytoplasm and small nuclei lacking prominent nucleoli), increased proliferative activity, and associated necrosis. The investigators emphasized that the tumor that they were describing was not a new entity but one that had likely been recognized in 1907 by Langerhans as *wuchernde Struma*[13] and subsequently regarded as a subset of various other diagnostic groups, including FTC, PTC, medullary thyroid carcinoma (MTC), and ATC.[10] Thus, PDTC as defined by Carcangiu and colleagues was a considerably more exclusive category compared with that of Sakamoto and colleagues, requiring high-grade features (mitotic activity and necrosis) in addition to a particular growth pattern.

Over the subsequent years, there was significant controversy in the thyroid pathology community about PDTC as a diagnostic entity.[14,15] In addition to the question of whether PDTC could be defined by growth pattern alone or required high-grade features as well, some groups were characterizing variants of PTC, such as tall cell and columnar cell variants, as PDTC on the basis of their more aggressive clinical behavior compared with conventional PTC.[16–18] Additionally, some studies were reporting a lack of prognostic significance of solid growth or an insular architecture alone.[19–21] Volante and colleagues[22] aimed to investigate the importance of high-grade features in tumors with a solid/trabecular/insular growth pattern. Examining a cohort of 183 cases with

these growth patterns (comprising at least 10% of the tumor), the investigators found that patient age, mitotic count greater than 3 per 10 high-power fields (HPFs), and tumor necrosis were all independent prognostic variables in multivariate analysis. Hiltzik and colleagues[7] further emphasized the importance of high-grade features. These investigators defined PDTC as a follicular cell–derived tumor that had tumor necrosis and/or greater than or equal to 5 mitoses per 10 HPFs, regardless of the tumor growth pattern. Of their cohort that included 58 patients, 66% patients had or developed distant metastases (predominantly lung and bone, with rare liver, spleen, and kidney metastases), 74% developed disease recurrence or disease progression, and 38% of patients died of disease, with a 5-year overall survival rate of 60%. Necrosis was present in 83% of cases and the mean mitotic rate was 6 mitoses per 10 HPFs. Although they reported that growth pattern did not seem to influence outcome, it should be noted that there was a predominant solid/trabecular/insular growth pattern in 79% of their cases.

It was not until 2004 that PDTC was recognized as a separate tumor entity in the World Health Organization (WHO) Tumors of Endocrine Organs.[23] In the 2004 WHO classification, PDTC was defined as a tumor with a predominantly solid/trabecular/insular architecture together with an infiltrative growth pattern, necrosis, and obvious vascular invasion. Additionally, the tumor cells of PDTC were described as generally small and uniform with hyperchromatic to vesicular nuclei and indistinct nucleoli. Importantly, tall cell and columnar cell variants of PTC were excluded from the category of PDTC. Although the 2004 WHO classification identified the main diagnostic features of PDTC, there was still uncertainty about how to apply the criteria and variability in application between pathologists in different countries. Hence, in 2006, an international consensus conference of 12 thyroid pathologists from Japan, Europe, and the United States was held in Turin, Italy; 83 cases from these countries that had areas of solid/trabecular/insular growth were reviewed.[5] Based on the review of these cases, an algorithmic approach was proposed for the diagnosis of PDTC. According to the Turin proposal, the diagnosis of PDTC requires the presence of a solid/trabecular/insular architecture, a lack of nuclear features of PTC, and the presence of one of the following: convoluted nuclei, necrosis, and/or a mitotic count of 3 or more per 10 HPFs. This approach was based on the finding that necrosis was strongly correlated with a shorter survival (regardless of extent), as was a mitotic count of 3 or more mitoses per 10 HPFs (although to a lesser extent than necrosis). Based on this approach, they showed that PDTCs had an outcome intermediate between well-differentiated thyroid carcinomas and ATC. Additionally, they found that there was no prognostic difference between PDTC with and without an associated PTC component. Although the investigators considered the presence of a solid/trabecular/insular pattern as sine qua non for the diagnosis of PDTC, and one or a combination of these architectures constituted 50% or more of the tumor in a majority of their cases, a cutoff value for the amount of tumor showing poorly differentiated features required to render a diagnosis of PDTC was not put forth. Additionally, oncocytic tumors were not included in the study, although the investigators suggested that similar criteria could likely be applied.

After the publication of the Turin proposal, a few studies were published that picked up where the Turin study left off. Dettmer and colleagues[6] aimed to evaluate what percentage of a tumor needs to show poorly differentiated features for it to be regarded as PDTC. To do this, they identified 42 cases that had an adverse clinical outcome (recurrent disease or death) and compared this group to a control group of 50 FTCs. For each case they evaluated the extent of the poorly differentiated component as defined by the Turin proposal using increments of 10%. They found 83% of the cases with an adverse outcome had a poorly differentiated component (89% of which had tumor necrosis). The poorly differentiated component comprised 50% or more of the tumor in 28 (80%) of the 35 cases, and it accounted for less than 50% in 7 (20%) cases. Tumors with a poorly differentiated component amounting to at least 10% of the tumor had significantly worse outcome by Kaplan-Meier analysis compared with those in the control group (they evaluated overall survival, tumor-specific survival, and relapse-free survival). Moreover, there was no difference in survival between groups with a poorly differentiated area of 10% to less than 50% and those with a poorly differentiated area of 50% or more. Finally, in multivariate analysis, a poorly differentiated area of at least 10% was the only consistent prognostically significant factor. Although these findings are helpful, the method in which cases were selected for the study could potentially introduce bias. In contrast, in a recent study by Gnemmi and colleagues,[4] they found that a solid/trabecular/insular architecture was significant for disease-free survival, but not cancer-specific survival, at a threshold of greater than or equal to 45% ($P = .0122$), with

the greatest significance at greater than or equal to 75% ($P = .0094$).

Although prior studies had reported oncocytic tumors that met Turin criteria for PDTC,[24] and in the 2004 WHO classification it was recognized that some PDTC have oncocytic features,[13] oncocytic tumors were excluded from the cohort of cases studied in Turin.[5] A subsequent study by Asioli and colleagues[1] confirmed, however, that utilization of the same diagnostic criteria was appropriate for oncocytic tumors. This study's methods are noteworthy: 1 of the investigators reviewed slides from 4570 primary thyroid malignancies that included 3128 resected at the Mayo Clinic between 1955 and 2000 and 1442 resected at 2 hospitals in Northern Italy between 1974 and 2008. As a result of this exhaustive review, the study's results are highly informative. They found that the prevalence of PDTC (defined by the Turin criteria, and with a well-differentiated component comprising <25% of the tumor) in the American cohort was 1.8% and in the Italian cohort was 6.7%. The higher prevalence in Northern Italy is consistent with a higher incidence of PDTC in areas with iodine deficiency. The mean age of the patients with PDTC in their cohort was 61, and the female-to-male ratio was 1.6 to 1. The 5-year survival for patients with PDTC was 71.6% and the 10-year survival was 46.3%. A mitotic count of greater than or equal to 3 per 10 HPFs was present in 94% of cases, 70% had necrosis, 10% had an associated well-differentiated PTC component, 24% had an associated well-differentiated FTC component, and significantly 32% were characterized as having greater than 75% oncocytic features. They found that oncocytic PDTC had a similar outcome to that of non-oncocytic PDTC. In a second study by Dettmer and colleagues,[3] these investigators also evaluated whether the Turin criteria could be applied to oncocytic tumors. They evaluated thyroid tumors from 129 patients with an adverse clinical outcome (recurrent disease or death) operated on between 1990 and 2006 and identified 16 conventional and 18 oncocytic tumors that were categorized as PDTC based on the Turin proposal (with at least 10% of the tumor comprised of a poorly differentiated component). In contrast to the findings of Asioli and colleagues, they found that patients with oncocytic PDTC did worse than those with conventional PDTC in terms of overall survival and tumor-specific survival (and this difference was maintained in multivariate analysis). They found there was no difference in relapse-free survival. Based on their findings and the result of another study that demonstrated that fewer than 10% of onco-cytic FTCs accumulate radioactive iodine com-pared with 75% of conventional FTCs,[25] the investigators postulated that the decrease in sur-vival for oncocytic PDTC compared with conven-tional PDTC may be secondary to decreased responsiveness to radioactive iodine treatment. Thus, the results of Dettmer and colleagues sug-gest that the presence of oncocytic features may have both prognostic and treatment implications. Although the studies by Asioli and colleagues and Dettmer and colleagues showed somewhat different results, they both demonstrated that the presence of oncocytic features should not alter the diagnostic algorithm for PDTC.

RENDERING A DIAGNOSIS OF POORLY DIFFERENTIATED THYROID CARCINOMA

MICROSCOPIC FEATURES

When evaluating whether a thyroid carcinoma is poorly differentiated, it is general consensus to start by evaluating whether the tumor has a solid/trabecular/insular growth pattern (**Fig. 1**). Although solid is used as a descriptor for the archi-tecture of PDTC, PDTCs with a solid architecture often do not have sheets of cells; rather, there is a vaguely nested architecture secondary to the capillary network within the tumor. Additionally, in areas of solid/trabecular/insular growth, there can be occasional small microfollicles. In PDTCs that do not demonstrate an entirely solid/trabec-ular/insular growth pattern, it is helpful to notice that along with a shift in architecture, there is a shift in cytomorphology, with a decrease in cell size and an increase in the nuclear to cytoplasmic ratio that can usually be appreciated even at low power (**Fig. 2**). The cells in PDTC are small and uniform (**Fig. 3A**). The nuclear-to-cytoplasmic ratio is high because the cells have scant eosinophilic cytoplasm. The nuclei of PDTC are uniform, small, and dark and may be convoluted (see **Fig. 3B**). That is, the nuclei have irregular nuclear contours reminiscent of the nuclei of PTC. In contrast to PTC, however, the nuclei are smaller, there is less nuclear clearing, grooves are less prominent, and the nuclear pseudoinclusions and the small marginalized nucleoli of PTC are absent. Once it is established that the tumor has areas of solid/trabecular/insular growth and lacks nuclear fea-tures of PTC in these areas, then the tumor should be examined for the presence of necrosis and/or a mitotic count of greater than or equal to 3 mitoses per 10 HPFs to establish the diagnosis of PDTC according to the Turin criteria (the presence of convoluted nuclei alone is discussed later). The

necrosis of PDTC is coagulative necrosis; hence, in the area of necrosis, the outlines of tumor cells that were previously viable (**Fig. 4**) can still be seen. Necrosis secondary to fine-needle aspira-tion (especially common in oncocytic tumors) must be excluded. A mitotic count should be generated using the area of highest mitotic activ-ity. Often the area of highest mitotic activity is adjacent to the areas of tumor necrosis. Some PDTCs are oncocytic (**Fig. 5**). These tumors are composed of cells with abundant granular eosi-nophilic cytoplasm with round nucleoli and prominent central nucleoli. Sometimes the nucleoli are not as prominent as they are in well-differentiated oncocytic neoplasms, with the chromatin appearing more clumped or coarse. As indicated in the previous discussion, the same criteria should be used when evaluating whether an oncocytic tumor is poorly differentiated. When rendering a diagnosis of PDTC, the term, *insular carcinoma*, should not be used because insular describes architecture alone, whereas the term PDTC reflects all of the aforementioned diagnostic criteria. Also, all of the histologic features that led to the diagnosis of PDTC (architecture, nuclear features, presence of necrosis, and the mitotic count per 10 HPFs) should be documented in the pathology report.

IMMUNOHISTOCHEMISTRY

Immunohistochemistry is not required to render a diagnosis of PDTC; however, staining may be used to support the diagnosis. PDTCs are positive for PAX8, TTF-1, and thyroglobulin. Compared with well-differentiated tumors, TTF-1 and thyroglobulin staining is generally weaker in PDTCs (**Fig. 6**).[5] Additionally, the thyroglobulin staining often has a dotlike paranuclear pattern (see **Fig. 6**).[1,5] Although this thyroglobulin staining pattern is characteristic of PDTC, it is not entirely specific because it has been observed in other benign and malignant thy-roid lesions with a predominantly solid/trabecular pattern.[5] Well-differentiated thyroid tumors have been shown to be negative for p53 immunohisto-chemical staining (<5% of tumor cells positive).[26] One group reported that a majority of cases of PDTC showed some p53 positivity and approxi-mately half showed diffuse positivity; however, a second group reported only focal staining in 30% of their cohort.[1,27] Although the reason for these conflicting results is unclear (both groups were us-ing Turin criteria), it can be concluded that whereas p53 immunohistochemical staining may support a diagnosis of PDTC, negative staining does not exclude the diagnosis. Moreover, focal p53 stain-ing (without an underlying p53 mutation) has been

Fig. 1. Growth patterns of PDTC: (*A*) solid (H&E stain), (*B*) trabecular (H&E stain), and (*C*) insular growth (H&E stain).

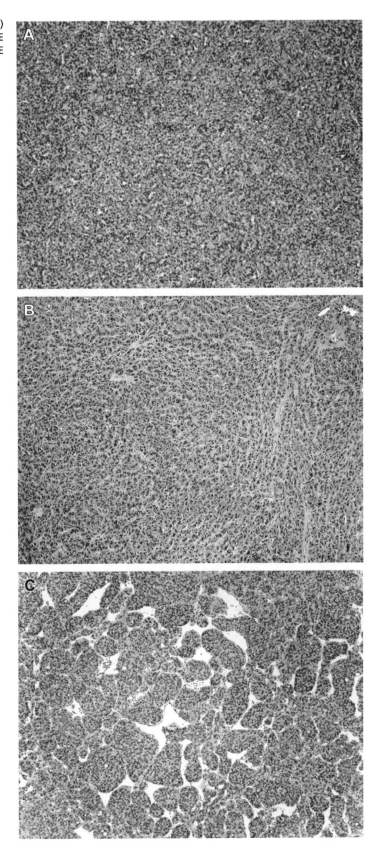

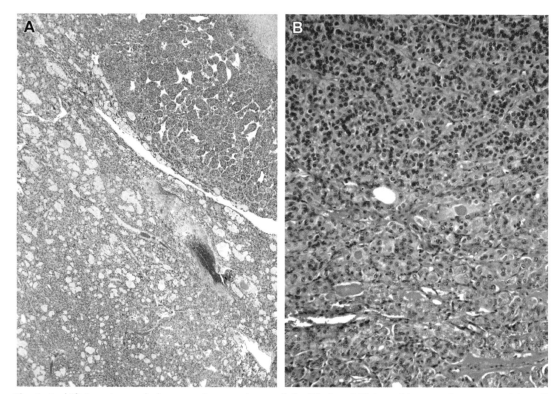

Fig. 2. A shift in cytomorphology can be seen in parallel with the shift in architecture in tumors with well-differentiated and poorly differentiated components (A) at low and at (B) high power (H&E stain).

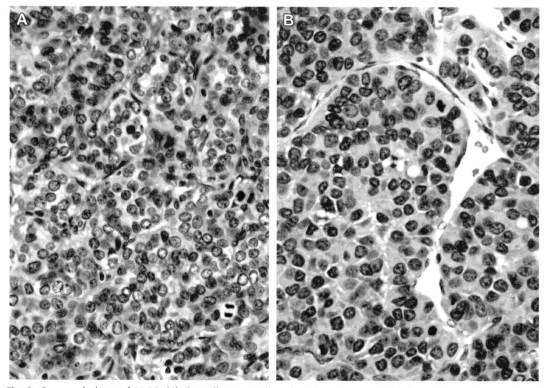

Fig. 3. Cytomophology of PDTC: (A) the cells are small and uniform (H&E stain) (B) nuclei may be convoluted (H&E stain).

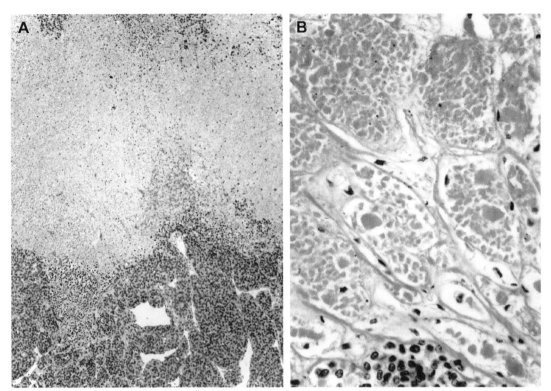

Fig. 4. Necrosis present within PDTC (*A*) at low and (*B*) at high power with outlines of previously viable tumor cells evident (H&E stain).

reported in some well-differentiated thyroid carcinomas.[28] Ki67 proliferative index has been reported to be below 5% in 95% of well-differentiated thyroid carcinomas.[26] The Ki67 index has been evaluated in 2 cohorts of PDTCs diagnosed according to Turin criteria; 1 group reported a mean Ki67 proliferative index of 13% (range 3%–40%), whereas the second group reported a mean Ki67 proliferative index of 3.7% (range 2%–10.7%).[1,4] Hence, again although an increased Ki67 index (above 5%) is supportive of a diagnosis of PDTC, not all PDTCs have a high Ki67 proliferative index. Additionally, rare well-differentiated tumors and aggressive PTC variants may have Ki67 proliferative index above 5%. The lack of sensitivity of increased Ki67 staining is not surprising given that some PDTCs may be diagnosed as such on the basis of necrosis and not increased mitotic activity.

DIFFERENTIAL DIAGNOSIS

SOLID VARIANT OF PAPILLARY THYROID CARCINOMA

Tumors with a solid architecture with nuclear features of PTC should be diagnosed as solid variant of PTC and not PDTC. In addition to the different nuclear characteristics that distinguish solid variant of PTC from PDTC, the cells of solid variant of PTC are significantly larger due to the fact that they have more eosinophilic cytoplasm. Thus, on low power, the tumors seem more eosinophilic overall compared with PDTC (Fig. 7A). On high power, the nuclei are larger, clearer, show more overlapping, and have more prominent grooves than PDTC (see Fig. 7B). The distinction is significant because although the solid variant of PTC has been associated with a slightly higher frequency of distant metastases and a less favorable prognosis than classical PTC, it is not associated the same aggressive clinical course as PDTC.[29] Increased mitotic activity and necrosis have been described in some cases of solid variant of PTC.[5,29] Although these findings do not indicate that the tumor is PDTC, they should be noted in the pathology report because necrosis and increased mitotic activity are prognostically significant findings.

AGGRESSIVE VARIANTS OF PAPILLARY THYROID CARCINOMA

In the study by Gnemmi and colleagues,[4] the investigators compared the utility of the Turin criteria and the criteria put forth by Hiltzik and

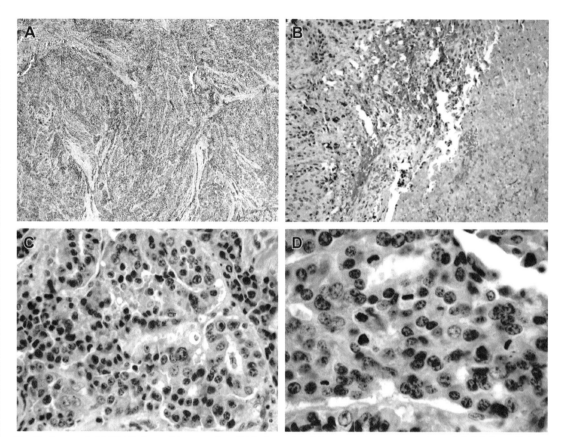

Fig. 5. Oncocytic PDTC (*A*) the architecture is solid (H&E stain), (*B*) necrosis is present (H&E stain), (*C*) the cells have abundant granular cytoplasm and nuclei with prominent nucleoli (H&E stain), and (*D*) mitotic activity is high (H&E stain).

colleagues (with PDTC defined solely on the basis of a mitotic count of ≥5 or necrosis) in a series of 82 thyroid carcinomas. Concordance between the Turin proposal and Hiltzik criteria was 75%. In general, some cases that would be classified as PDTC by the Hiltzik criteria on the basis of increased mitotic activity and necrosis are likely to be aggressive PTC variants, such as columnar cell and hobnail cell variant (**Fig. 8**). Although these tumors have been shown to pursue an aggressive clinical course,[18,30] there is general consensus in the literature that these should be recognized as PTC variants and not PDTC.

MEDULLARY THYROID CARCINOMA

Both PDTC and MTC can have a solid/nested/insular growth pattern, a monomorphic appearance, and a lack of associated colloid. Additionally, not all MTCs have associated amyloid deposition, and the salt-and-pepper chromatin of MTC may not be obvious if there is crush artifact. Therefore, MTC may enter into the differential diagnosis when considering the diagnosis of

PDTC (**Fig. 9**). In general, MTCs have a lower nuclear-to-cytoplasmic ratio than PDTC and usually do not have increased mitotic activity or necrosis. If there is any question histologically, immunohistochemistry should be performed. Both MTC and PDTC are positive for TTF-1 and PAX8. MTCs are positive, however, for calcitonin (almost always), mCEA, synaptophysin, and chromogranin, whereas PDTCs are negative for these stains. In contrast, PDTCs usually demonstrate at least some degree of staining for thyroglobulin whereas thyroglobulin staining is negative in MTCs.

ANAPLASTIC THYROID CARCINOMA

ATC and PDTC are both associated with increased mitotic activity and necrosis. However, ATCs are markedly pleomorphic compared with PDTCs (**Fig. 10**), the cells and nuclei of ATC are generally much larger than those of PDTC, and many ATCs demonstrate a spindle cell or squamoid morphology that is not seen with PDTC. Additionally, the mitotic count of ATC is higher than that of

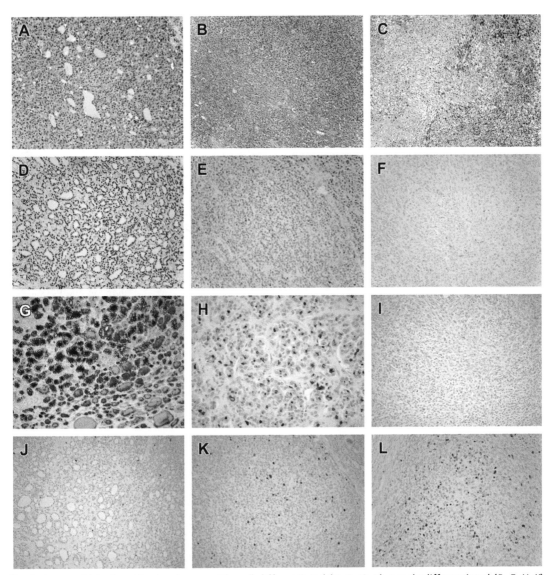

Fig. 6. Immunohistochemistry in a tumor with well-differentiated (*A, D, G, H*), poorly differentiated (*B, E, H, K*), and anaplastic (*C, F, I, L*) components: TTF-1 expression (*D, E, F*) is reduced in the poorly differentiated areas and lost the anaplastic component. Thyroglobulin staining (*G, H, I*) is reduced in the poorly differentiated area (and shows the characteristic dot-like paranuclear pattern) and lost in the anaplastic component. Ki67 expression (*J, K, L*) is almost absent in the well-differentiated component, increased in the poorly differentiated component, and highest in the anaplastic component.

PDTC, and atypical mitoses are more frequently present. For PDTC diagnosed by Turin criteria, a mean mitotic count of 1.9 to 5 per 10 HPFs has been reported, with atypical mitoses seen in 20% of cases,[1,3,4] whereas, for ATC, mitoses are typically abundant (it is not unusual to see 5 mitoses in a single HPF) and atypical mitoses are present in almost all cases. Immunohistochemistry can also help differentiate ATC from PDTC. Although PDTCs usually demonstrate some positivity for thyroglobulin, expression is almost always lost in ATC (see **Fig. 7**). Also, TTF-1 staining is markedly reduced (if present) in ATC (see **Fig. 7**), the Ki67 proliferative index is much higher (usually approximately 50%–60%) in ATC (see **Fig. 7**), and keratin expression is significant reduced in ATC compared with PDTC.[31,32] Some PDTCs may show progression to ATC. Recognition of an ATC component is important because tumors with even a small area of ATC can pursue a rapidly fatal course.[5]

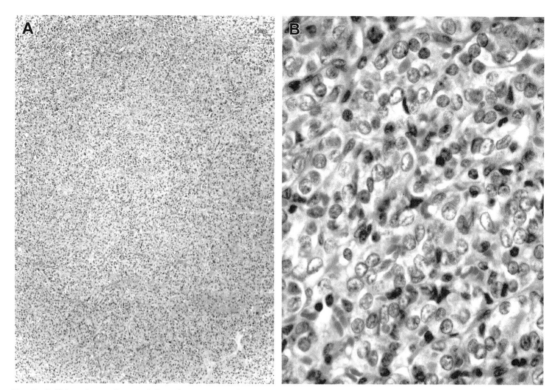

Fig. 7. Solid variant of PTC: (*A*) at low power the low nuclear to cytoplasmic ratio compared with that seen in PDTC can be appreciated (H&E stain); (*B*) at high power the characteristic nuclear features of PTC can be appreciated, including nuclear enlargement, overlapping, clearing, contour irregularities, and grooves (H&E stain).

UNRESOLVED ASPECTS OF THE DIAGNOSIS OF POORLY DIFFERENTIATED THYROID CARCINOMA

Although considerable progress has been made in establishing the definition of PDTC, there are still aspects of the diagnosis that call for of additional investigation.[33–36] Probably the most problematic point is that of the convoluted nuclei of PDTC. Although it is clear that many PDTCs have convoluted nuclei, it is unclear whether convoluted nuclei along with a solid/trabecular/insular component are sufficient for a diagnosis of PDTC as put forth in the Turin proposal.[5] A vast majority of reported cases of PDTC with convoluted nuclei diagnosed using Turin criteria have also had a mitotic count of greater than or equal to 3 mitoses per 10 HPFs or tumor necrosis.[1,4–6] Moreover, in the subsequent studies by Asioli and colleagues[1] and Gnemmi and colleagues,[4] convoluted nuclei failed to provide prognostic value. And, as noted by Sadow and Faquin,[33] assessment of convoluted nuclei may be a subjective challenge. Thus, it is questionable whether a tumor with a solid/trabecular/insular architecture and a lack of

nuclear features of PTC should be characterized as PDTC on the basis of convoluted nuclei alone. Because of these issues, for the rare cases with solid/trabecular/insular growth pattern and convoluted nuclei alone, the senior author of this review would not render a diagnosis of PDTC but instead document the histologically worrisome features in a note. A second unresolved issue is the percentage of tumor showing poorly differentiated features that is required to consider a tumor as PDTC. Although the study by Dettmer and colleagues[6] suggests that a diagnosis of PDTC could be justified when at least 10% of the tumor has poorly differentiated features, other investigators have required a much higher percentage,[1] demonstrating a lack of consensus in the literature on this point. Although it may not be established what the top-line diagnosis of tumors with focal poorly differentiated features should be, based on the results of Dettmer and colleagues study it seems clear that the histologic findings should be documented in the pathology report in some manner. Finally, in the 2004 WHO classification, PDTC was defined as an infiltrative tumor with obvious vascular invasion.[6] Although infiltrative growth and vascular invasion were not overtly stated

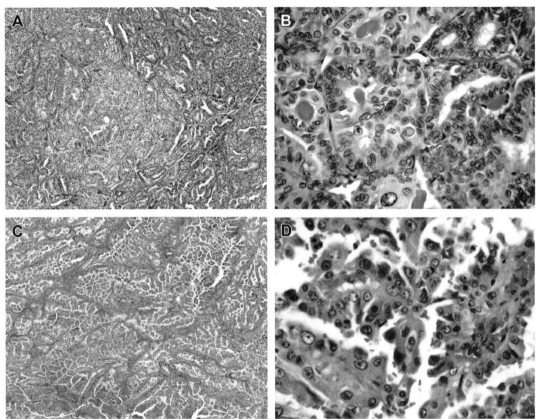

Fig. 8. Aggressive variants of PTC: columnar cell variant (*A*, *B*) and hobnail cell variant (*C*, *D*) (H&E stain).

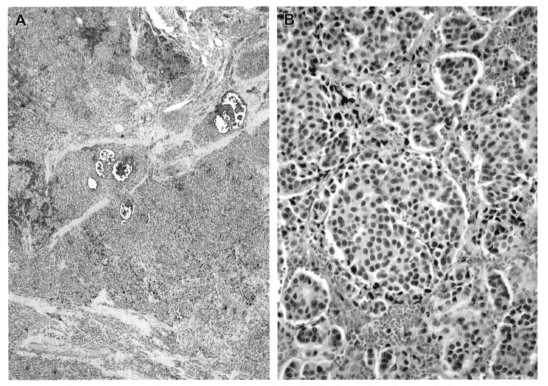

Fig. 9. MTC: (*A*) at low power the growth pattern and lack of colloid could result in confusion with PDTC (H&E stain); (*B*) at higher power the nuclear to cytoplasmic ratio is lower than expected for PDTC (H&E stain).

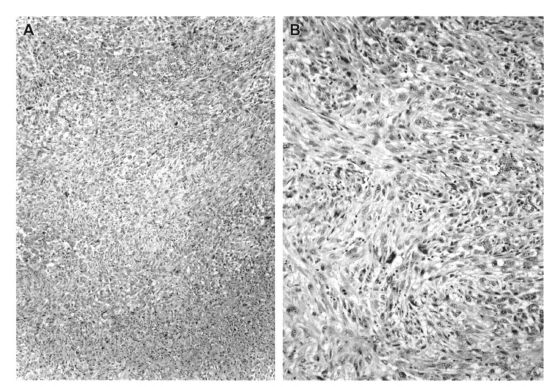

Fig. 10. ATC at low (*A*) and high (*B*) power. In contrast to the small, uniform cells of PDTC, ATC typically shows striking pleomophism and marked cytologic atypia (H&E stain).

criteria for PDTC according to the Turin proposal, vascular invasion was present in 92% of the cases that were scored for vascular invasion in that series, and in the Turin validation study lymphovascular invasion was present in 99% of cases.[1,5] The few cases reported in the literature of encapsulated tumors with high-grade features without capsular penetration or lymphovascular invasion pursued an indolent clinical course,[37] indicating that such tumors should not be diagnosed as PDTC. Additional studies evaluating the clinical outcome of encapsulated tumors and tumors with focal capsular penetration alone (ie, without lymphovascular invasion) with necrosis and increased mitotic activity are warranted.[33]

MOLECULAR ALTERATIONS OF POORLY DIFFERENTIATED THYROID CARCINOMA

Approximately 70% of well-differentiated thyroid carcinomas harbor a known genomic alteration, including point mutations in *BRAF* and RAS family members and rearrangements involving *RET/PTC* and *PAX8/PPARγ*.[38] The most common mutations in PTCs are activating *BRAF* mutations and RAS family member mutations (RAS mutations are

seen in follicular variant of PTC), with rarer *RET/PTC* and *PAX8/PPARγ* rearrangements.[39] FTCs lack *BRAF* mutations and *RET/PTC* translocations; instead, they most frequently harbor RAS mutations, with rarer *PAX8/PPARγ* rearrangements.[40–45] Much of the molecular data reported prior to the Turin criteria are difficult to interpret because of the highly heterogeneous classification criteria.[46] In a study performed after the Turin proposal, Volante and colleagues[27] screened 65 cases of PDTC for RAS family and *BRAF* mutations and *RET/PTC* and *PAX8/PPARγ* rearrangements. They found RAS family mutations in 15 (23%) of 65 cases (which were evenly distributed between nononcocytic and oncocytic PDTCs), with 14 *NRAS* mutations (Q61R) and 1 *HRAS* mutation (Q61K). Only 1 case (a PDTC with an associated PTC component) harbored a *BRAF*V600E mutation. No cases had *KRAS* mutations or *RET/PTC* or *PAX8/PPARγ* rearrangements. More than 70% of the cases in their cohort had no identifiable mutation. An association with RAS family mutations and relatively infrequent *BRAF* mutations has been reported in other studies evaluating the molecular alterations of PDTC.[45–48] If further studies confirm these results, they have interesting implications in terms of the tumorigenesis of PDTCs. For one, the fact that many PDTCs appear to lack the common mutations/rearrangements seen in well-differentiated thyroid carcinomas suggests that many PDTCs are either arising de novo or arising from well-differentiated thyroid carcinomas without the common molecular alterations reported in these tumors. The higher frequency of RAS family mutations compared with *BRAF* mutations suggests that more PDTCs may be related to FTC or follicular variant of PTC than classical type PTC. The low percentage of *BRAF* mutations found in PDTC compared with ATC[48] could indicate that when *BRAF*-mutant PTCs progress, they progress straight to ATC or progress quickly through a poorly differentiated state. Finally, the paucity of *RET/PTC* and *PAX8/PPAR*γ rearrangements in PDTCs suggest that well-differentiated tumors harboring these alterations may be less predisposed to dedifferentiation.[49]

Additional mutations reported in PDTC that are thought to occur late in tumorigenesis (ie, they are not seen in well-differentiated thyroid carcinomas) include *TP53* mutations and β-catenin gene mutations. *TP53* mutations have been reported in approximately 25% of PDTCs[28,50] and may underlie the increased chromosomal instability seen in PDTC compared with well-differentiated tumors.[49,51] The results for β-catenin gene mutations have been conflicting. Although 1 group reported β-catenin gene mutations in 25% (with concomitant Wnt signaling activation), a second group failed to find any mutations in their cohort of PDTCs.[52] There is still much to learn about the genetic and epigenetic events that underlie PDTC. Hopefully future studies that use techniques that allow for more comprehensive interrogation of PDTCs will uncover additional molecular alterations.

REFERENCES

1. Asioli S, Erickson LA, Righi A, et al. Poorly differentiated carcinoma of the thyroid: validation of the Turin proposal and analysis of IMP3 expression. Mod Pathol 2010;23(9):1269–78.

2. Ito Y, Hirokawa M, Fukushima M, et al. Prevalence and prognostic significance of poor differentiation and tall cell variant in papillary carcinoma in Japan. World J Surg 2008;32(7):1535–43 [discussion: 1544–5].

3. Dettmer M, Schmitt A, Steinert H, et al. Poorly differentiated oncocytic thyroid carcinoma–diagnostic implications and outcome. Histopathology 2012; 60(7):1045–51.

4. Gnemmi V, Renaud F, Do Cao C, et al. Poorly differentiated thyroid carcinomas: application of the Turin proposal provides prognostic results similar to those from the assessment of high-grade features. Histopathology 2014;64(2):263–73.

5. Volante M, Collini P, Nikiforov YE, et al. Poorly differentiated thyroid carcinoma: the Turin proposal for the use of uniform diagnostic criteria and an algorithmic diagnostic approach. Am J Surg Pathol 2007;31(8):1256–64.

6. Dettmer M, Schmitt A, Steinert H, et al. Poorly differentiated thyroid carcinomas: how much poorly differentiated is needed? Am J Surg Pathol 2011; 35(12):1866–72.

7. Hiltzik D, Carlson DL, Tuttle RM, et al. Poorly differentiated thyroid carcinomas defined on the basis of mitosis and necrosis: a clinicopathologic study of 58 patients. Cancer 2006;106(6): 1286–95.

8. Pellegriti G, Giuffrida D, Scollo C, et al. Long-term outcome of patients with insular carcinoma of the thyroid: the insular histotype is an independent predictor of poor prognosis. Cancer 2002;95(10): 2076–85.

9. Buckwalter JA, Nordschow CD. A moot thyroid neoplasm: carcinoma or sarcoma. Ann Surg 1958; 148(1):115–8.

10. Rosai J, Saxen EA, Woolner L. Undifferentiated and poorly differentiated carcinoma. Semin Diagn Pathol 1985;2(2):123–36.

11. Sakamoto A, Kasai N, Sugano H. Poorly differentiated carcinoma of the thyroid. A clinicopathologic entity for a high-risk group of papillary and follicular carcinomas. Cancer 1983;52(10):1849–55.

12. Carcangiu ML, Zampi G, Rosai J. Poorly differentiated ("insular") thyroid carcinoma. A reinterpretation of Langhans' "wuchernde Struma". Am J Surg Pathol 1984;8(9):655–68.

13. Langhans T. Über die epithelialen Formen der malignen Struma. Virchows Arch (path Anat) 1907;189:69–188.

14. Akslen LA, LiVolsi VA. Poorly differentiated thyroid carcinoma–it is important. Am J Surg Pathol 2000; 24(2):310–3.

15. Albores-Saavedra J, Carrick K. Where to set the threshold between well differentiated and poorly differentiated follicular carcinomas of the thyroid. Endocr Pathol 2004;15(4):297–305.

16. Nishida T, Katayama S, Tsujimoto M, et al. Clinicopathological significance of poorly differentiated thyroid carcinoma. Am J Surg Pathol 1999;23(2): 205–11.

17. Pilotti S, Collini P, Manzari A, et al. Poorly differentiated forms of papillary thyroid carcinoma: distinctive entities or morphological patterns? Semin Diagn Pathol 1995;12(3):249–55.

18. Sobrinho-Simoes M, Nesland JM, Johannessen JV. Columnar-cell carcinoma. Another variant of poorly differentiated carcinoma of the thyroid. Am J Clin Pathol 1988;89(2):264–7.

19. Akslen LA, Myking AO, Salvesen H, et al. Prognostic importance of various clinicopathological features in papillary thyroid carcinoma. Eur J Cancer 1992;29A(1):44–51.

20. Ashfaq R, Vuitch F, Delgado R, et al. Papillary and follicular thyroid carcinomas with an insular component. Cancer 1994;73(2):416–23.

21. Carcangiu ML, Zampi G, Pupi A, et al. Papillary carcinoma of the thyroid. A clinicopathologic study of 241 cases treated at the University of Florence, Italy. Cancer 1985;55(4):805–28.

22. Volante M, Landolfi S, Chiusa L, et al. Poorly differentiated carcinomas of the thyroid with trabecular, insular, and solid patterns: a clinicopathologic study of 183 patients. Cancer 2004; 100(5):950–7.

23. DeLellis RA. Pathology and genetics of tumours of endocrine organs. Lyon (France): IARC Press; 2004.

24. Papotti M, Torchio B, Grassi L, et al. Poorly differentiated oxyphilic (Hurthle cell) carcinomas of the thyroid. Am J Surg Pathol 1996;20(6):686–94.

25. Yutan E, Clark OH. Hurthle cell carcinoma. Curr Treat Options Oncol 2001;2(4):331–5.

26. Saltman B, Singh B, Hedvat CV, et al. Patterns of expression of cell cycle/apoptosis genes along the spectrum of thyroid carcinoma progression. Surgery 2006;140(6):899–905 [discussion: 905–6].

27. Volante M, Rapa I, Gandhi M, et al. RAS mutations are the predominant molecular alteration in poorly differentiated thyroid carcinomas and bear prognostic impact. J Clin Endocrinol Metab 2009; 94(12):4735–41.

28. Dobashi Y, Sugimura H, Sakamoto A, et al. Stepwise participation of p53 gene mutation during dedifferentiation of human thyroid carcinomas. Diagn Mol Pathol 1994;3(1):9–14.

29. Nikiforov YE, Erickson LA, Nikiforova MN, et al. Solid variant of papillary thyroid carcinoma: incidence, clinical-pathologic characteristics, molecular analysis, and biologic behavior. Am J Surg Pathol 2001;25(12):1478–84.

30. Asioli S, Erickson LA, Sebo TJ, et al. Papillary thyroid carcinoma with prominent hobnail features: a new aggressive variant of moderately differentiated papillary carcinoma. A clinicopathologic, immunohistochemical, and molecular study of eight cases. Am J Surg Pathol 2010;34(1):44–52.

31. Nikiforov Y. Diagnostic pathology and molecular genetics of the thyroid. 2nd edition. Philadelphia: Wolters Kluwer/Lippincott Williams & Wilkins Health; 2012.

32. Erickson LA, Jin L, Wollan PC, et al. Expression of p27kip1 and Ki-67 in benign and malignant thyroid tumors. Mod Pathol 1998;11(2):169–74.

33. Sadow PM, Faquin WC. Poorly differentiated thyroid carcinoma: an incubating entity. Front Endocrinol (Lausanne) 2012;3:77.

34. Sanders EM Jr, LiVolsi VA, Brierley J, et al. An evidence-based review of poorly differentiated thyroid cancer. World J Surg 2007;31(5):934–45.

35. Volante M, Papotti M. Poorly differentiated thyroid carcinoma: 5 years after the 2004 WHO classification of endocrine tumours. Endocr Pathol 2010; 21(1):1–6.

36. Volante M, Rapa I, Papotti M. Poorly differentiated thyroid carcinoma: diagnostic features and controversial issues. Endocr Pathol 2008;19(3):150–5.

37. Rivera M, Ricarte-Filho J, Patel S, et al. Encapsulated thyroid tumors of follicular cell origin with high grade features (high mitotic rate/tumor necrosis): a clinicopathologic and molecular study. Hum Pathol 2010;41(2):172–80.

38. Nikiforov YE. Molecular diagnostics of thyroid tumors. Arch Pathol Lab Med 2011;135(5):569–77.

39. Jung CK, Little MP, Lubin JH, et al. The increase in thyroid cancer incidence during the last four decades is accompanied by a high frequency of BRAF mutations and a sharp increase in RAS mutations. J Clin Endocrinol Metab 2014;99(2): E276–85.

40. Dwight T, Thoppe SR, Foukakis T, et al. Involvement of the PAX8/peroxisome proliferator-activated receptor gamma rearrangement in follicular thyroid tumors. J Clin Endocrinol Metab 2003;88(9):4440–5.

41. Ezzat S, Zheng L, Kolenda J, et al. Prevalence of activating ras mutations in morphologically characterized thyroid nodules. Thyroid 1996;6(5):409–16.

42. Karga H, Lee JK, Vickery AL Jr, et al. Ras oncogene mutations in benign and malignant thyroid neoplasms. J Clin Endocrinol Metab 1991;73(4): 832–6.

43. Marques AR, Espadinha C, Catarino AL, et al. Expression of PAX8-PPAR gamma 1 rearrangements in both follicular thyroid carcinomas and adenomas. J Clin Endocrinol Metab 2002;87(8): 3947–52.

44. Nikiforova MN, Biddinger PW, Caudill CM, et al. PAX8-PPARgamma rearrangement in thyroid tumors: RT-PCR and immunohistochemical analyses. Am J Surg Pathol 2002;26(8):1016–23.

45. Nikiforova MN, Lynch RA, Biddinger PW, et al. RAS point mutations and PAX8-PPAR gamma rearrangement in thyroid tumors: evidence for distinct molecular pathways in thyroid follicular carcinoma. J Clin Endocrinol Metab 2003;88(5):2318–26.

46. Basolo F, Pisaturo F, Pollina LE, et al. N-ras mutation in poorly differentiated thyroid carcinomas: correlation with bone metastases and inverse correlation to thyroglobulin expression. Thyroid 2000;10(1): 19–23.

47. Pilotti S, Collini P, Mariani L, et al. Insular carcinoma: a distinct de novo entity among follicular carcinomas of the thyroid gland. Am J Surg Pathol 1997;21(12):1466–73.

48. Soares P, Trovisco V, Rocha AS, et al. BRAF mutations typical of papillary thyroid carcinoma are more frequently detected in undifferentiated than in insular and insular-like poorly differentiated carcinomas. Virchows Arch 2004;444(6):572–6.

49. Soares P, Lima J, Preto A, et al. Genetic alterations in poorly differentiated and undifferentiated thyroid carcinomas. Curr Genomics 2011;12(8):609–17.

50. Donghi R, Longoni A, Pilotti S, et al. Gene p53 mutations are restricted to poorly differentiated and undifferentiated carcinomas of the thyroid gland. J Clin Invest 1993;91(4):1753–60.

51. Wreesmann VB, Ghossein RA, Patel SG, et al. Genome-wide appraisal of thyroid cancer progression. Am J Pathol 2002;161(5):1549–56.

52. Rocha AS, Soares P, Fonseca E, et al. E-cadherin loss rather than beta-catenin alterations is a common feature of poorly differentiated thyroid carcinomas. Histopathology 2003;42(6): 580–7.

Immunohistochemical Diagnosis of Thyroid Tumors

Guido Fadda, MD, MIAC*, Esther Diana Rossi, MD, MIAC, PhD

KEYWORDS
- Thyroid carcinoma • Immunochemistry • Prognosis • Target therapy

ABSTRACT

Recent insight into the molecular mechanisms of thyroid carcinogenesis has led to studies involving newly directed antibodies. With the introduction of new molecular targeted therapies, these antibodies may represent useful predictors of therapeutic response in tumors unresponsive to radioiodine or insensitive to conventional antitumor therapies. These markers complement the development of markers that are able to discern benign from malignant entities, including hyalinizing trabecular tumors, oncocytic neoplasms, and follicular variant of papillary thyroid carcinoma. The use of antibodies directed to proteins generated by mutated genes may represent a cost-effective method for diagnosing and managing patients affected by thyroid tumors.

OVERVIEW

Thyroid neoplasms represent the most common endocrine tumors, with an incidence of 8.7 cases/100,000 people per year in Europe, although overall mortality is less than 0.1% in all tumor cases[1,2]

The classification of thyroid neoplasms[3] includes benign and malignant epithelial tumors derived from either follicular cells or parafollicular common (C) cells. Papillary thyroid carcinoma (PTC) is the most thyroid cancer, accounting for almost 90% of all thyroid malignancies, often with a favorable course characterized by frequent nodal spreading but uncommon distant metastases. PTC includes 2 main tumor subtypes: classical type and follicular variant. The former exhibits the distinctive papillary structures from which the name derives whereas the histologic hallmark of the latter is the predominantly microfollicular pattern, lacking true papillae. Regardless of the architecture, the diagnosis of PTC relies on distinctive nuclear features (clearing, elongation, grooves, and pseudoinclusions), which are usually shared by all histotypes, the latter rarer in the follicular variant.

Some cases of PTC show obvious infiltration of surrounding tissues in addition to either invasion of an associated tumor capsule or the adjacent vessels, manifesting the malignant nature of the tumor. On the other hand, some cases, of follicular variant, for instance, are encapsulated and lack invasion, and the histologic definition of carcinoma can be questionable.

Thyroid epithelial malignancies include follicular thyroid carcinoma (FTC), approximately 5% of thyroid carcinomas, characterized by a proliferation of follicular cells (thyrocytes) showing variably pleomorphic and variably chromatic nuclei. The distinction between FTC and its benign counterpart, follicular adenoma (FA), relies on the detection of histologic parameters of invasion, capsular and/or vascular invasion. If only one of such features is observed in a follicular-patterned, nonpapillary neoplasm, a diagnosis of FTC is warranted. These parameters for malignancy apply similarly to tumors composed exclusively of Hürthle (or oxyphilic or oncocytic) cells, FTC, and oncocytic (Hürthle cell) type (Hurthle cell carcinoma [HCC]), with oncocytic changes thought to result from hypoxic changes of the thyrocytes. FTC and HCC are more likely to metastasize to distant sites, such as lung and bone, rather than the local lymph node and neck involvement seen in PTC.

The authors do not have conflicts of interest to disclose.

Division of Anatomic Pathology and Histology, Agostino Gemelli School of Medicine and Hospital, Catholic University, Largo Francesco Vito, Rome 1 00168, Italy

* Corresponding author.

E-mail address: guidofadda@rm.unicatt.it

http://dx.doi.org/10.1016/j.path.2014.08.002
1875-9181/14/$ – see front matter

Other thyrocyte-derived malignancies include poorly differentiated thyroid carcinoma (PDTC) and undifferentiated (anaplastic) thyroid carcinoma (ATC). They represent no more than 3% of all thyroid carcinomas and the majority of thyroid-related mortalities. Of the nonfollicular thyroid malignancies, the most important are medullary thyroid carcinoma (MTC) and non-Hodgkin lymphoma.

IMMUNOHISTOCHEMISTRY

Immunohistochemistry (IHC) was introduced in the early 1970s into routine pathology practice. It has been traditionally used in thyroid pathology for the identification of the cell origin in differentiated tumors arising in the gland or metastasizing outside it, such as thyroglobulin, calcitonin, or parathyroid hormone.[4] There are some tumor types which immunophenotyping deserves a more detailed discussion. Hyalinizing trabecular tumors (HTTs) are uncommon neoplasms with morphology that overlaps that of PTC. HTT exhibits a trabecular pattern with hyalinization of the stroma composed of thyrocytes showing intranuclear pseudoinclusions resembling those of PTC and, in some cases, RET/PTC rearrangements.[5,6] This tumor, however, is generally of low malignant potential.[7] Leonardo and colleagues[8] have proposed an immunohistochemical method for differentiating HTT from PTC. Namely, cytoplasmic (membranous) expression of MIB-1 antibody, directed toward the cell-cycle protein Ki-67, instead of nuclear expression of Ki-67, which is used as proliferative index in many tumors. The unusual experimental conditions (room temperature instead of 37°C) and the strict histologic criteria for diagnosing pure forms have somewhat hindered the diffusion of this diagnostic marker.

Hürthle cell tumors (HCTs) (or oxyphilic and oncocytic tumors) are included in the category of follicular thyroid tumors, although they do not share all of its histologic characteristics. Hürthle cells, thought to be a metaplastic change of thyrocytes due to either local hypoxia or hormone withdrawal, show a distinctive morphology, with large pleomorphic nuclei and abundant granular cytoplasm which, at the ultrastructural level, is rich in mitochondria and responsible for the oncocytic features of HC seen by hematoxylineosin stain and, by IHC, for the mild nonspecific positivity of these cells in a majority of IHC reactions. Thus, the real positivity of Hürthle cells should be assessed only in presence of a strong expression in the majority of the cellular component (like thyroglobulin usually does) or when the antibody expression is primarily nuclear (like

thyroid transcription factor-1 [TTF-1]). The IHC stains that are helpful in the other differentiated tumors (such as galectin-3, Hector Battifora mesothelial antigen [HBME-1], and cytokeratin [CK] 19; discussed later) provide controversial results in HCT and are regarded as unreliable for discriminating benign from malignant neoplasms. Some studies involving HCT have reported that some proliferative markers, such as Ki-67 and cyclin D1, may be of help in this differential diagnosis.[9] A different approach to oncocytic tumors has been studied by Gasparre and colleagues.[10] They have observed that the oncocytic metaplasia, originated by a marked increase of the mitochondrial component in the cytoplasm of the follicular cells, is often associated with a nonsense mutation of the ND-5 subunit of the respiratory chain complex I of the mitochondria. The expression of the human mitochondrial antibody (HMA) against this subunit reveals the presence of oncocytic cells, regardless of their malignant nature. In this case, the HMA does not represent a marker of malignancy but, nonetheless, this is an important parameter to take into account for a diagnosis of follicular-patterned neoplasm because oncocytic cells sometimes are misdiagnosed as PTC cells. The diagnosis of PTC does not require capsular or vascular invasion, unlike oncocytic carcinomas, which are diagnosed on the basis of invasion. Thus, the expression of HMA in a wholly encapsulated follicular neoplasm favors the diagnosis of benign oncocytic adenoma whereas its negativity suggests a papillary carcinoma.

Medullary thyroid carcinoma can be easily distinguished from follicular neoplasms by calcitonin expression. Cytoplasmic calcitonin expression, however, may be weak or the antibody may leak in the normal parenchyma, hindering the correct interpretation of the morphologic picture, especially when the tumor is of small size or in presence of a C-cell hyperplasia. Usually, C cells show a concomitant bright, albeit nonspecific, positivity for carcinoembryonic antigen, chromogranin A, bombesin, synaptophysin, and other neuroendocrine markers.[4] Recently, aquaporins (AQPs) 3 and 4 have been investigated in MTC in comparison with differentiated follicular-derived tumors showing a distinct pattern of expression: AQP-4 exhibits the same positivity as thyroglobulin whereas AQP-3 results distinctively negative in PTC and FA and positive in the cytoplasm membrane of C cells.[11]

ATCs lose the distinctive immunophenotype of follicular-derived thyroid carcinomas, such as the expression of thyroglobulin and TTF-1. Diagnosis of ATC relies mainly on tumor morphology with nonspecific cytoplasmic expression of low- and high-molecular-weight CKs. Another important diagnostic marker is p53 (**Fig. 1**), which is often overexpressed in a majority of nuclei of ATC and represents an important marker for this tumor because it is less prolific in differentiated and PDTC.[12] Although the infrequency of ATC does not justify the introduction of specific antibodies for the undifferentiated cells, one recent study has focused on the expression of cancer stem cell markers (protein associated with embryonic development [SOX-2], ATP-binding cassette [ABC], CXCR4, multidrug resistance associated protein 1 [MRP-1], and lung resistance protein [LRP] antibodies) in this tumor versus differentiated carcinomas with the perspective of using these antibodies as prognostic or predictive markers[13] (discussed later).

IMMUNOMARKERS OF MALIGNANCY

One of the greatest challenges in thyroid pathology is differentiation between benign and malignant follicular-patterned neoplasms.[14] The traditional identification of features of aggressiveness of the tumor capsule and its surrounding structures (normal parenchyma, vessels, and skeletal muscle) is the pivotal criterion on which this distinction is founded. Although some cases of PTC do not exhibit these features, nuclear features of PTC warrant a diagnosis of malignancy. A few cases of encapsulated lesions exhibiting a follicular structure, however, either do not show nuclear features of PTC in a large amount of cells or display only focal nuclear clearing and irregularity, which do not allow for a reliable diagnosis of malignancy. IHC markers of malignancy, which may distinguish malignant from benign lesions irrespective of the histologic features of carcinomatous transformation (especially capsular or vascular invasion), have, in recent years, been a frequently availed adjuvant to the morphologic diagnosis of thyroid cancer.[15] HBME-1, originally produced for being applied in the discrimination between mesothelioma and adenocarcinoma of the lung, has been one of the first antibodies to be used for the diagnosis of thyroid carcinoma.[16] Since then, more than 20 antibodies have been tested with the hope of superceding or at least complementing nuclear features of the thyrocytes. A recent article by Correia Rodrigues and colleagues[17] has evaluated the clinical results of 25 antibodies that have been tested in approximately 100 different studies on thyroid fine-needle aspiration, and similar findings were registered by Griffith and coworkers.[15] The most studied markers of malignancy are HBME-1, galectin-3, and CK19. Apart from HBME-1, whose epitope in the microvilli of the mesothelial is still unknown, the others are well characterized molecules: for example, galectin-3 is a member of the lectin family, molecules that recognize and bind β-galactoside residues in glycoproteins and glycolipids, which have extensively been studied in histologic and cytologic samples.[18–20] CK19 is a low-molecular-weight intermediate filament of the cytoplasm, which has also been extensively studied (**Box 1**).[21,22]

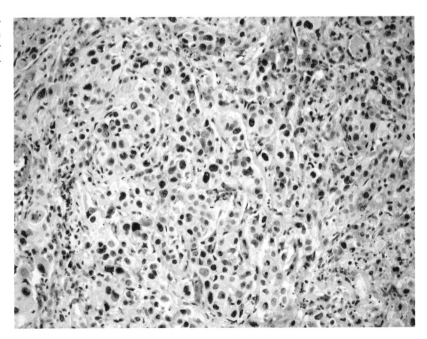

Fig. 1. High rate of nuclear positivity of an anaplastic carcinoma for p53 (ABC, original magnification ×125).

Each of the antibodies discussed previously exhibits a characteristic expression pattern that may be helpful in some diagnostic settings. HBME-1 membranous staining (**Fig. 2**) is specific for the malignant thyrocytes and is often useful in identifying microcarcinomas as small as a few millimeters. Galectin-3 shows strong cytoplasmic positivity (**Fig. 3**), which is most sensitive compared with HBME-1 expression but may be detected in benign cells with clear cytoplasm. It also marks vascular smooth muscle, which can be used as internal positive controls. CK19 exhibits a strong cytoplasmic expression (**Fig. 4**), prominent in neoplastic cells but often with positive expression in benign thyrocytes.[22] Many studies have focused on the reliability of each of these antibodies to distinguish benign from malignant neoplasms on both histologic formalin-fixed paraffin-embedded (FFPE) sections and fine-needle aspiration biopsy material. The unanimous conclusion has been that no single antibody achieves such a high accuracy for being used in this crucial diagnostic task. Thus, the best combination of these antibodies and others (discussed later) has been investigated with the aim of harmonizing the high positive predictive value of CK19 and HBME-1 with the high negative predictive value of galectin-3. According to the review of Griffith and colleagues,[15] the best results on FFPE sections were obtained with the panel made up of CK19, galectin-3, and HBME-1 with different combinations of 2 of them. De Matos and colleagues,[23] in their large series of thyroid neoplasms, reported good sensitivity (84%–96.5%) and diagnostic accuracy (DA) (84.9%) for the combination of the 3 markers in the diagnosis of PTC whereas the same parameters resulted significantly lower for FTC (63.1%). Similar results were obtained by Park and colleagues,[24] Scognamiglio and colleagues,[25] and Rossi and colleagues,[26] using different combinations of the antibodies discussed previously, reporting a DA of greater than 90%. A recent article by Nechifor-Boila and colleagues[27] has investigated the accuracy of a panel of 4 antibodies (HBME-1, galectin-3, CK19, and CD56) in providing the correct discrimination between malignant and benign

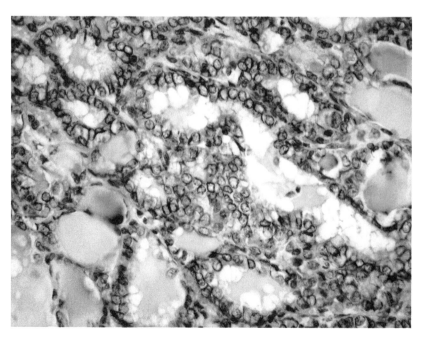

Fig. 2. Membranous positivity of HBME-1 in a follicular variant of papillary carcinoma (ABC, original magnification ×250).

Fig. 3. Cytoplasm positivity of galectin-3 in a follicular variant of PTC (ABC, original magnification ×250).

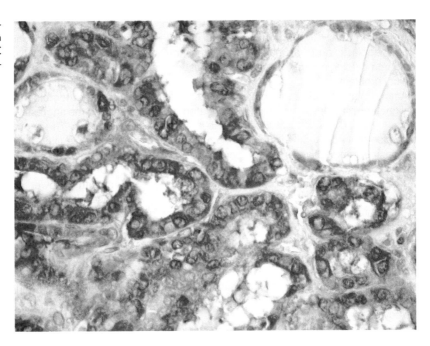

follicular neoplasms. Their results do not support the use of a combination of more than 3 antibodies, especially when the diagnosis concerns the follicular variant of PTC. In the review by Correia Rodrigues and colleagues,[17] galectin-3 has proved the most reliable and effective malignancy marker in both FFPE and cytologic materials followed by HBME-1, thyroperoxidase (TPO), and CK19. These investigators, evaluating many studies, concluded that although galectin-3 shows on average a positive predictive value and negative predictive value of, respectively, 84.1% and 81% and a DA of approximately 83%, these results were not sufficient for recommending the use of this antibody alone for the differential diagnosis between malignant and benign neoplasms. Nonetheless, in the

Fig. 4. Intense cytoplasm positivity of CK19 in a classic variant of PTC (ABC, original magnification ×400).

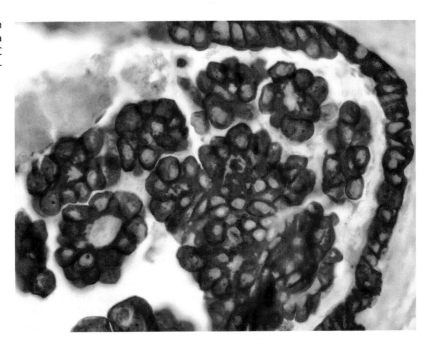

field of thyroid cytology, galectin-3, especially in combination with HBME-1, may be helpful in identifying neoplastic and malignant lesions in the indeterminate cytologic categories, which represent a clinical problem.[28–30]

Among the antibodies that have been tested as malignancy markers in thyroid differentiated tumors, TPO, CD57, CD44v6, and Rb-1[27,31,32] have also proved effective in identifying malignant neoplasms irrespective of the presence of either capsular or vascular invasion, although the results are controversial because of the poor reproducibility of some experiments (TPO and Rb1).

There are some recently investigated markers of malignancy that have revealed good accuracy in identifying the malignant cells of a follicular-patterned neoplasm. FGFR-2 is an isoform of the fibroblast growth factor receptor family and is underexpressed in PTC and FA whereas it exhibits strong cytoplasmic expression in normal and hyperplastic thyrocytes.[33] The retinoic acid receptors (RARs) and the retinoid X receptors (RXRs), each including 2 isoforms A and B, have shown good sensitivity (RARs) and specificity (RXRs) in PTCs. It is remarkable that the expression of these antibodies is different in malignant and benign cells, the latter with strong nuclear expression and the former identified by a marked cytoplasmic staining.[34]

The malignancy markers have been also studied in other thyroid tumors.[35] In these instances the IHC does not focus on the identification of malignant cells, because the histologic hallmarks of malignancy are usually well detectable but on the correct recognition of the poorly differentiated component, which can be important for the prognosis and the treatment of the tumor.

PROGNOSTIC AND PREDICTIVE MARKERS

The IHC expression of antibodies that may either anticipate the degree of aggressiveness or predict the clinical course of a malignant tumor has long been investigated. Traditional proliferative markers, such as Ki-67, p27/kip1, and cyclins D1 and E, have been tested first in the differential diagnosis of malignant versus benign differentiated tumors, then as prognostic parameters in the same neoplastic category with controversial results.[36–38]

Wang and colleagues[39] have suggested that a score based on the expression of the connective tissue growth factor, also known as CCN2, may predict with high statistical significance the possibility of a high tumor stage at diagnosis and the likelihood of regional nodal metastases. Similar results were reported by Saffar and colleagues,[40] who tested matrix metalloprotease (MMP) 2 and caspase (CCP) 3 in PTC. MMP2 did not show a significant correlation with necrosis or extrathyroid extension but was significantly associated with a higher likelihood of lymphatic spread, whereas CCP3 showed a specular correlation with the same prognostic parameters. The investigators suggest the combined use of both antibodies for assessing the aggressiveness of PTC for therapeutic purposes. The expression of neural cell adhesion molecule (NCAM) (CD56) and ovarian cancer immunoreactive antigen domain containing 1 (OCIAD-1) in thyroid differentiated tumors is associated with a lower aggressiveness whereas a decreased or absent positivity in the neoplastic cells may be predictive of nodal or distant metastatic spread; in a few cases, the metastatic thyrocytes retrieve the expression of CD56.[41]

More interesting are the recent investigations leading to the application of prognostic markers to less differentiated and undifferentiated tumors, especially ATC, for which new pharmacologic treatments (sorafenib, axitinib, and withaferin A) with monoclonal antibodies directed against the growth factor receptors of the neoplastic cells have been recently introduced.[42,43] In this setting, the expression of cancer stem cell markers, discussed previously,[13] has been associated with a worse clinical course and may be evaluated in patients who are candidates for targeted therapies.

PDTC is an uncommon finding in routine practice, usually observed by its growth pattern in the context of a differentiated carcinoma. Nevertheless, many investigators have reported a decrease of the disease-free interval and of the overall survival in tumors showing a predominantly insular growth pattern (usually >40% of the tumor volume). Recently, an article by Rossi and colleagues[35] found, in a small series of pure insular carcinomas, a statistically significant correlation with the expression of nucleus-localized β-catenin compared with more traditional malignancy markers (HBME-1 and galectin-3) in PTC.

MARKERS OF GENE MUTATIONS

The recent discoveries of the involvement of the most important signaling pathways of the follicular cells in the thyroid carcinogenesis have led the investigation of the role of each single gene mutation in the cell transformation. As a consequence, studies investigating mutations in the genes involved in the MAP kinase signaling cascade have provided brilliant data supporting the pivotal importance of RAF and RAS mutations in the origin of thyrocyte-related carcinomas as well as point mutations of *RET* regarded as key for the development of MTC.[44–46] Many of these investigations have been carried out at molecular level but, as a

Fig. 5. Marked positivity of PTC for the BRAF VE-1 antibody (ABC, original magnification ×50).

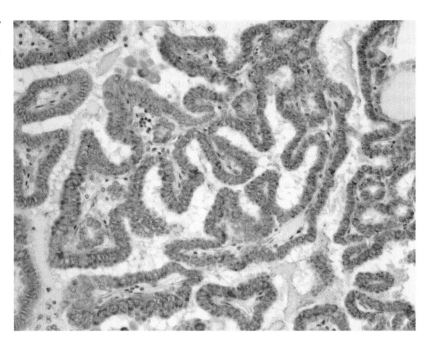

natural consequence, some antibodies directed toward the mutated proteins have been produced and released for different clinical purposes.

RET proto-oncogene, an antibody with cytoplasm expression, was used at the beginning of this century as a malignancy marker for follicular differentiated tumors.[15,26] Unfortunately, because of technical problems and a significant lack of specificity, its application for this important differential diagnosis has been discontinued in most institutions.

For similar reasons, use of PAX8/PPARgamma antibody, which was regarded as a robust diagnostic marker of FTC,[47,48] also showed significant positive expression in FA (31%),[49] hampering its diagnostic utility.

More recently, an antibody directed toward the BRAF mutated protein kinase (VE-1) has become commercially available as a diagnostic and prognostic marker.[50] Its expression, according to investigators who have published on this subject, would reveal the presence of the V600E mutation of *BRAF*, the most commonly identified genetic mutation in PTC.[45,46,51] The identification of a *BRAF* mutation can be helpful in 2 different clinical settings: (1) on cytologic material when an indeterminate diagnosis is made on a fine-needle aspiration biopsy and (2) on both cytologic and FFPE materials, when the diagnosis of PTC is already evident (**Fig. 5**). In the former case, *BRAF* mutation is regarded as 99% specific for PTC, identifying those patients who should be directed toward total

thyroidectomy and sparing many unnecessary thyroid removals. In the second scenario, preoperative cytologic or postlobectomy for completion for known PTC, the identification of *BRAFV600E* mutation would provide surgeons with an additional tool for a more aggressive approach to either the tumor or the central neck compartment nodes.[52]

Rossi and colleagues[53] also imply that in aspiration samples cytologically suspicious for PTC, with 60% to 80% likelihood for PTC diagnosis at excision, the identification of a *BRAF* mutation might render a more aggressive surgical approach.

The most important condition for the use of the antibody VE-1 as a morphologic substitute of the molecular change is the nearly complete overlap between molecular and IHC findings.[54]

SUMMARY

Recent insight into the molecular mechanisms of thyroid carcinogenesis has led to a flourishing of studies involving newly directed antibodies. With the introduction of new molecular targeted therapies, these new antibodies may represent useful predictors of therapeutic response in tumors unresponsive to radioiodine or insensitive to conventional antitumor therapies (primarily surgery), such as PDTCs, ATCs, and well-differentiated carcinomas that are not surgically resectable or have metastasized. These markers complement the development of markers that, at their best clinical use, are able to discern benign from malignant entities, including HTT, oncocytic neoplasms, and follicular variant of PTC. Although several IHC biomarkers have been reported in small studies in recent years, their efficacy has yet to be validated. Finally, the use of antibodies directed to proteins generated by mutated genes may represent a cost-effective method for diagnosing and managing patients affected by thyroid tumors.

REFERENCES

1. Hundahl SA, Cady B, Cunningham MP, et al. Initial results from a prospective cohort study of 5583 cases of thyroid carcinoma treated in the united states during 1996. U.S. and German Thyroid Cancer Study Group. An American College of Surgeons Commission on Cancer Patient Care Evaluation study. Cancer 2000;89(1):202–17.

2. Gimm O. Mini-review: thyroid cancer. Canc Lett 2001;163:143–56.

3. De Lellis RA, Lloyd RV, Heitz PU, et al. World Health Organisation pathology and genetics of tumours of endocrine organs. Lyon (France): IARC press; 2004. p. 49–123. Agency for Research on Cancer.

4. Khan A, Nosè V. Pathology of the thyroid gland. In: Lloyd RV, editor. Endocrine pathology. Totowa (NJ): Humana Press; 2004.

5. Carney JA, Hirokawa M, Lloyd RV, et al. Hyalinizing trabecular tumors of the thyroid gland are almost all benign. Am J Surg Pathol 2008;32(12):1877–89.

6. Cheung CC, Boerner SL, MacMillan CM, et al. Hyalinizing trabecular tumor of the thyroid: a variant of papillary carcinoma proved by molecular genetics. Am J Surg Pathol 2000;24(12):1622–6.

7. Papotti M, Volante M, Giuliano A, et al. RET/PTC activation in hyalinizing trabecular tumors of the thyroid. Am J Surg Pathol 2000;24(12):1615–21.

8. Leonardo E, Volante M, Barbareschi M, et al. Cell membrane reactivity of MIB-1 antibody to Ki67 in human tumors: fact or artifact? Appl Immunohistochem Mol Morphol 2007;15:220–3.

9. Erickson LA, Jin L, Goellner JR, et al. Pathologic features, proliferative activity, and cyclin D1 expression in Hurthle cell neoplasms of the thyroid. Mod Pathol 2000;13(2):186–92.

10. Gasparre G, Porcelli AM, Bonora E, et al. Disruptive mitochondrial DNA mutations in complex I subunits are markers of oncocytic phenotype in thyroid tumors. Proc Natl Acad Sci U S A 2007;104(21):9001–6.

11. Niu D, Kondo T, Nakazawa T, et al. Differential expression of aquaporins and its diagnostic utility in thyroid cancer. PLoS One 2012;7(7):e40770.

12. Gauchotte G, Philippe C, Lacomme S, et al. BRAF, p53 and SOX2 in anaplastic thyroid carcinoma: evidence for multistep carcinogenesis. Pathology 2011;43(5):447–52.

13. Yun JY, Kim YA, Choe JY, et al. Expression of cancer stem cell markers is more frequent in anaplastic thyroid carcinoma compared to papillary thyroid carcinoma and is related to adverse clinical outcome. J Clin Pathol 2014;67(2):125–33.

14. Baloch ZW, LiVolsi VA. Follicular-patterned lesions of the thyroid: the bane of the pathologist. Am J Clin Pathol 2002;117:143–50.

15. Griffith OL, Chiu CG, Gown AM, et al. 2008 Biomarker panel diagnosis of thyroid cancer: a critical review [review]. Expert Rev Anticancer Ther 2008;8:1399–413.

16. Miettinen M, Kovatich AJ. HBME-1 monoclonal antibody useful in the differential diagnosis of mesothelioma, adenocarcinoma and soft tissue and bone tumors. Appl Immunohistochem 1995;3: 115–22.

17. Correia Rodrigues HG, de Pontes AA, Adan LF. Use of molecular markers in samples obtained from preoperative aspiration of thyroid [review]. Endocr J 2012;59(5):417–24.

18. Bartolazzi A, Gasbarri A, Papotti M, et al. Application of an immunodiagnostic method for improving preoperative diagnosis of nodular thyroid lesions. Lancet 2001;357:1644–50.

19. Papotti M, Volante M, Saggiorato E, et al. Role of galectin-3 immunodetection in the cytological diagnosis of thyroid cystic papillary carcinoma. Eur J Endocrinol 2002;147:515–21.

20. Herrmann ME, LiVolsi VA, Pasha TL, et al. Immunohistochemical expression of Galectin-3 in benign and malignant thyroid lesions. Arch Pathol Lab Med 2002;126:710–3.

21. Dencic TI, Cvejic D, Paunovic I, et al. Cytokeratin19 expression discriminates papillary thyroid carcinoma from other thyroid lesions and predicts its aggressive behavior. Med Oncol 2013;30:362–71.

22. Sahoo S, Hoda SA, Rosai J, et al. Cytokeratin 19 immunoreactivity in the diagnosis of papillary thyroid carcinoma: a note of caution. Am J Clin Pathol 2001;116(5):696–702.

23. De Matos LL, Del Giglio AB, Matsubayashi CO, et al. Expression of CK-19, galectin-3 and HBME-1 in the differentiation of thyroid lesions: systematic review and diagnostic meta-analysis [review]. Diagn Pathol 2012;7:97.

24. Park YJ, Kwak SH, Kim DC, et al. Diagnostic value of galectin-3, HBME-1, cytokeratin 19, high molecular weight cytokeratin, cyclin D1 and p27(kip1) in the differential diagnosis of thyroid nodules. J Korean Med Sci 2007;22(4):621–8.

25. Scognamiglio T, Hyjek E, Kao J, et al. Diagnostic usefulness of HBME1, galectin-3, CK19, and CITED1 and evaluation of their expression in encapsulated lesions with questionable features of papillary thyroid carcinoma. Am J Clin Pathol 2006;126(5):700–8.

26. Rossi ED, Raffaelli M, Mule' A, et al. Simultaneous immunohistochemical expression of HBME-1 and galectin-3 differentiates papillary carcinomas from hyperfunctioning lesions of the thyroid. Histopathology 2006;48:795–800.

27. Nechifor-Boila A, Borda A, Sassola A, et al. Immunohistochemical markers in the diagnosis of papillary thyroid carcinomas: the promising role of combined immunostaining using HBME-1 and CD56. Pathol Res Pract 2013;209:585–92.

28. Rossi ED, Raffaelli M, Minimo C, et al. Immunocytochemical evaluation of thyroid neoplasms on thin-layer smears from fine-needle aspiration biopsies. Cancer 2005;105:87–95.

29. Saggiorato E, De Pompa R, Volante M, et al. Characterization of thyroid "follicular neoplasms" in fine-needle aspiration cytologic specimens using a panel of immunohistochemical markers: a proposal for clinical application. Endocr Relat Cancer 2005; 12:305–17.

30. Fadda G, Rossi ED, Raffaelli M, et al. Follicular thyroid neoplasms can be classified as low and high risk according to HBME-1 and Galectin 3 expression on liquid based fine needle cytology. Eur J Endocrinol 2011;165:447–53.

31. Anwar F, Emond MJ, Schmidt RA, et al. Retinoblastoma expression in thyroid neoplasms. Mod Pathol 2000;13:562–9.

32. Nasir A, Catalano E, Calafati S, et al. Role of p53, CD44V6 and CD57 in differentiating between benign and malignant follicular neoplasms of the thyroid. In Vivo 2004;18:189–95.

33. Redler A, Di Rocco G, Giannotti D, et al. Fibroblast growth factor receptor-2 expression in thyroid tumor progression: potential diagnostic application. PLoS One 2013;8:e72224.

34. Gauchotte G, Lacomme S, Brochin L, et al. Retinoid acid receptor expression is helpful to distinguish between adenoma and well-differentiated carcinoma in the thyroid. Virchows Arch 2013; 462:619–32.

35. Rossi ED, Straccia P, Palumbo M, et al. Diagnostic and prognostic role of HBME-1, galectin-3, and β-catenin in poorly differentiated and anaplastic thyroid carcinomas. Appl Immunohistochem Mol Morphol 2013;21:237–41.

36. Erickson LA, Jin L, Wollan PC, et al. Expression of p27kip1 and Ki-67 in benign and malignant thyroid tumors. Mod Pathol 1998;11:169–74.

37. Wang S, Wuu J, Savas L, et al. The role of cell cycle regulatory proteins, cyclin D1, cyclin E, and p27 in thyroid carcinogenesis. Hum Pathol 1998;29: 1304–9.

38. Konturek A, Barczyński M, Nowak W, et al. Prognostic factors in differentiated thyroid cancer–a 20-year surgical outcome study. Langenbecks Arch Surg 2012;397:809–15.

39. Wang G, Zhang W, Meng W, et al. Expression and clinical significance of connective tissue growth factor in thyroid carcinomas. J Int Med Res 2013; 41:1214–20.

40. Saffar H, Sanii S, Emami B, et al. Evaluation of MMP2 and Caspase-3 expression in 107 cases of papillary thyroid carcinoma and its association with prognostic factors. Pathol Res Pract 2013; 209:195–9.

41. Yang AH, Chen JY, Lee CH, et al. Expression of NCAM and OCIAD1 in well-differentiated thyroid carcinoma: correlation with the risk of distant metastasis. J Clin Pathol 2012;65:206–12.

42. Denaro N, Nigro CL, Russi EG, et al. The role of chemotherapy and latest emerging target therapies in anaplastic thyroid cancer [review]. Onco Targets Ther 2013;9:1231–41.

43. Cohen SM, Mukerji R, Timmermann BN, et al. A novel combination of withaferin A and sorafenib shows synergistic efficacy against both papillary and anaplastic thyroid cancers. Am J Surg 2012; 204:895–900.

44. Soares P, Trovisco V, Rocha AS, et al. Braf mutations typical of papillary thyroid carcinoma are more frequently detected in undifferentiated than in insular and insular-like poorly differentiated carcinomas. Virchows Arch 2004;444:572–6.

45. Eszlinger M, Paschke R. Molecular fine-needle aspiration biopsy diagnosis of thyroid nodules by tumor specific mutations and gene expression patterns. Mol Cell Endocrinol 2010;322:29–37.

46. Xing M. Braf mutation in papillary thyroid cancer: pathogenic role, molecular bases, and clinical implications. Endocr Rev 2007;28:742–62.

47. Kroll TG, Sarraf P, Pecciarini L, et al. Pax8-PPAR-gamma1 fusion oncogene in human thyroid carcinoma. Science 2000;25(289):1357–60.

48. Nikiforova MN, Biddinger PW, Caudill CM, et al. Nikiforov YE PAX8-PPARgamma rearrangement in thyroid tumors: RT-PRC and immunohistochemical analyses. Am J Surg Pathol 2002;26:1016–23.

49. Marques AR, Espadhina C, Catarino AL, et al. Expression of PAX8-PPARgamma 1 rearrangements in both follicular thyroid carcinomas and adenomas. J Clin Endocrinol Metab 2002;87: 3947–52.

50. Koperek O, Kornauth C, Capper D, et al. Immunohistochemical detection of the BRAF V600E-mutated protein in papillary thyroid carcinoma. Am J Surg Pathol 2012;36:844–50.

51. Nikiforova MN, Nikiforov Y. Molecular diagnostics and predictors in thyroid cancer. Thyroid 2009;19: 1351–61.

52. Cooper DS, Doherty GM, Haugen BR, et al. Revised management guidelines for patients with thyroid nodules and differentiated thyroid cancer. Thyroid 2009;19:1167–214.

53. Rossi ED, Martini M, Capodimonti S, et al. Diagnostic and prognostic value of immunocytochemistry and BRAF mutation analysis on liquid based biopsies of thyroid neoplasms suspicious for carcinoma. Eur J Endocrinol 2013;168:853–9.

54. Ghossein RA, Katabi N, Fagin JA. Immunohistochemical detection of mutated BRAF V600E supports the clonal origin of BRAF-induced thyroid cancers along the spectrum of disease progression. J Clin Endocrinol Metab 2013;98:e1414–21.

Tumor-Associated Inflammatory Cells in Thyroid Carcinomas

Marc P. Pusztaszeri, MD[a],*, William C. Faquin, MD, PhD[b,c],
Peter M. Sadow, MD, PhD[b,c]

KEYWORDS

- Thyroid • Cancer • Inflammation • Dendritic cells • Macrophages • Mast cells • Lymphocytes
- Chemokine

ABSTRACT

The complex interactions between immune cells and tumor cells in cancer play a major role in tumor development and subsequent patient outcomes. Different types of tumor-associated inflammatory cells (TAICs), such as dendritic cells, macrophages, lymphocytes, and mast cells, have been recognized for many years in several tumors; however, the role of TAICs in cancer is still not completely understood. This review article focuses on the major types of TAICs, including their general role in cancer and, more specifically, their role and distribution in thyrocyte-derived carcinomas.

OVERVIEW

The link between cancer and inflammation was first proposed approximately 250 years ago with the observation by Rudolf Virchow (1821–1902), a German pathologist, that tumors in different organs often arose in sites of chronic inflammation, and that inflammatory cells, including macrophages, were present within and around tumors.[1] Classic examples include *Helicobacter pylori*–associated gastric cancer and inflammatory bowel disease–associated colorectal cancer. In the thyroid gland, an association between chronic lymphocytic thyroiditis (CLT) (Hashimoto or autoimmune thyroiditis) and papillary thyroid carcinoma (PTC) has been reported in several studies since the 1950s.[2–4] Although chronic inflammation is a well-known risk factor for tumor initiation and promotion, once established, cancer cells may also produce proinflammatory chemokines within the tumor bed, supporting cancer progression.[5,6] Simultaneously, cancer cells must also evade destruction by the immune system to persist and thrive, a recognized hallmark of cancers,[7] which frequently arise in a background of immunodeficiency.[8] Conversely, aspirin, the most prolific anti-inflammatory drug worldwide, has been shown to reduce the incidence and mortality of several cancers (eg, colorectal) and is being considered for daily prophylaxis.[9] Therefore, the complex interactions between immune cells and tumor cells play a major role in tumor development, including tumor growth, invasion and metastasis, and subsequent patient outcomes.

Tumor-associated inflammatory cells (TAICs), including dendritic cells (DCs), macrophages, lymphocytes, and mast cells (MCs), have been recognized for many years in several tumors,[6,10–16] where they can play both protumorigenic and antitumorigenic roles (Jekyll and Hyde role), depending on cell number, state of activation, and surrounding microenvironment. It has been suggested that dysfunction of DCs induced by the tumor is a critical mechanism for escaping immune surveillance in cancer.[17,18] The role of TAICs in cancer, however, is not fully understood.

The authors have nothing to disclose.
[a] Department of Pathology, Geneva University Hospital, 1 Michel-Servet St, Geneva, GE 1211, Switzerland;
[b] Department of Pathology, Massachusetts General Hospital, Warren 219, 55 Fruit Street, Boston, MA 02114, USA; [c] Harvard Medical School, 25 Shattuck St, Boston, MA 02115, USA
* Corresponding author. Service de Pathologie Clinique, Hôpitaux Universitaires de Genève, 1 rue Michel-Servet, Genève 14 1211, Switzerland.
E-mail address: Marc.Pusztaszeri@hcuge.ch

Surgical Pathology 7 (2014) 501–514
http://dx.doi.org/10.1016/j.path.2014.08.006
1875-9181/14/$ – see front matter © 2014 Elsevier Inc. All rights reserved.

In the thyroid gland, there are 4 primary types of thyrocyte-derived carcinomas: well-differentiated thyroid carcinomas (WDTCs), including PTC and follicular thyroid carcinoma (FTC), poorly differentiated thyroid carcinomas (PDTCs), and anaplastic thyroid carcinomas (ATCs). PTC is the most common thyroid malignancy (80%–90%), and it is usually associated with an excellent prognosis and therapeutic response, primarily surgical. However, 10% to 30% of PTC patients who have undergone primary thyroidectomy and radioiodine treatment develop recurrences and metastases, largely in regional lymph nodes, that are usually sensitive to further radiodine treatment. In contrast, ATC, the most aggressive form of thyroid carcinoma, has a dismal prognosis because patients with ATC are rarely candidates for surgery, and their tumor is typically resistant to conventional treatments. Therefore, there is a need for new treatment modalities, including targeted therapies and/or immunotherapies, mostly in patients with advanced and/or poorly differentiated cancers, where conventional treatments with surgery and radioiodine therapy are not (or no longer) effective.

On the genetic level, PTC harbors distinct molecular alterations that are mutually exclusive: the point mutations in the BRAF or (H, K, and N) RAS genes, and RET/PTC rearrangements. These genetic alterations are present in up to 70% of PTC cases, with BRAF mutation the most common (approximately 40% of PTCs),[19] and result in activation of the mitogen-activated protein kinase cascade. The oncoproteins expressed in PTC may trigger a proinflammatory program in tumor cells by release of cytokines/chemokines and/or upregulation of their receptors.[20–26] BRAF mutations and RET/PTC rearrangements are highly specific for PTC,[19] although they may also be present in a subset of ATCs that are probably derived from PTC. In contrast, RAS gene mutations can also be found in up to 40% of thyroid follicular adenomas (FAs).

This article focuses on the major types of TAICs, including their general role in cancer and, more specifically, their role and distribution in the major thyrocyte-derived carcinomas. The role of the TAIC-related immunomodulators (cytokines and chemokines) in thyroid cancer is also briefly discussed.

TUMOR-ASSOCIATED INFLAMMATORY CELLS

The cell population in any cancer, including thyroid cancer, is heterogeneous, not solely comprising neoplastic cells but also consisting of various amounts of fibroblasts, endothelial cells, and TAICs, depending on tumor type, size, stage, and prior treatment (Box 1).[7] In some cancers,

---

Box 1
Tumor-associated Inflammatory Cells in Thyroid Cancer

1. Different types of tumor-associated inflammatory cells are present in thyroid cancer.

2. Cancer cells attract inflammatory cells through the release of many chemokines.

3. These cells play a major role in thyroid cancer where they can be both protumorigenic or antitumorigenic.

4. In contrast to other thyroid cancers, papillary carcinoma is characterized by the presence of numerous intratumoral dendritic cells.

5. Anaplastic thyroid carcinoma is characterized by the presence of numerous intratumoral macrophages with peculiar morphology.

---

such as lymphoepithelial carcinoma or seminoma, neoplastic cells may be obscured by the reactive TAICs, which are composed mainly of T lymphocytes.[27,28] Tumor-infiltrating macrophages (TAMs) can represent up to 50% of the tumor mass in some cancers, including ATCs.[29,30] On the other hand, some of these TAICs are not apparent on routine microscopic examination and may require immunohistochemistry for detection and phenotypic characterization.[31] In general, pathologists tend to regard TAICs in cancer only as part of the background architecture or reactive milieu, with a main focus on the architectural, histologic, and cytologic features of the tumor proper, for diagnostic and prognostic reporting. Recent studies demonstrate that nonneoplastic elements, such as TAICs, may predict the clinical behavior of a cancer even better than the characteristics of the neoplastic cells themselves.[32]

DENDRITIC CELLS

DCs originate from hematopoietic precursors in the bone marrow and subsequently migrate to peripheral tissues where they mature. DCs are highly specialized (so-called professional) antigen-presenting cells that play a major role during the primary immune responses against pathogens and tumors.[10,33–35] After cytokine exposure, immature DCs, including Langerhans cells, migrate from peripheral tissues to lymphoid organs, where they participate in antigen-specific immune responses.[36,37] They subsequently lose their ability to capture and process antigens (including tumor antigens) and acquire the ability to stimulate naïve T cells. The interaction of DCs with naïve T cells can lead to increased effector T-cell responses and/or to T-cell tolerance, depending on the type of DCs (immunogenic vs tolerogenic) and their state of activation.[38,39] For example, the plasmacytoid type of DC (pDCs) has been reported to exhibit potent immunosuppressive and tolerogenic properties by blocking proliferation of naïve and antigen-specific CD4+ and CD8+ T cells and supporting activation of T-regulatory lymphocytes (Tregs).[40] In contrast, pDCs have also been shown to present antigens to cytotoxic T lymphocytes, inducing efficient immune responses.[41] In the thyroid gland, an increased number of pDCs was found in association with PTC, where they may control proliferation, differentiation, and function of Tregs,[39] thereby contributing to the immune escape of PTC.[40] In addition to modifying T-cell response, DCs also contribute to natural killer (NK) cell antitumoral function and to B-cell–mediated immunity, with evidence that DCs may also function as direct cytotoxic effectors against tumors (so-called killer DCs).[42]

Although TAMs and MCs are generally considered protumorigenic,[11,12,14] DCs may have a crucial role in the development of antitumor immunity[10,13,17,43] and are being actively studied for potential immunotherapy against cancer (DC-based vaccines).[17] Several studies have suggested a positive correlation between DC number and prolonged survival,[13,43,44] including in PTC,[44] but this association remains controversial.[45] Although a high number of tumor-infiltrating DCs may intuitively suggest a strong immune response against the tumor, the relationship is by far more complex. In patients with cancer and in animal tumor models, the DCs present in tumor tissues and draining lymph nodes are often functionally defective.[17,18,46] Some studies have demonstrated that tumor-infiltrating DCs lack costimulatory molecules and possess poor T-cell–stimulatory capacity or induce anergy.[47] Moreover, tumor-derived factors, such as vascular endothelial growth factor (VEGF), transforming growth factor (TGF)-β, and interleukin (IL)-10, can induce apoptosis of DCs, inhibit functional maturation of DCs, and convert DCs into tolerogenic DCs.[17,46] Therefore, DCs in cancer, including in PTC, usually have an immature phenotype with defective ability to stimulate T cells.[17,34] This may reflect lack of effective maturation signals or the presence of maturation inhibitors in the tumor microenvironment. Taken together, these data suggest that DCs are most likely poor inducers of immune responses to tumor antigens and that they may even mediate tolerance instead of immune activation.

DENDRITIC CELLS IN THE NORMAL THYROID GLAND AND IN PAPILLARY THYROID CARCINOMA

In the normal thyroid gland, DCs are rare or absent.[31,44,45,48,49] Compared with normal thyroid tissue and other thyroid tumors, including FTC, FA, Hürthle cell neoplasms, medullary thyroid carcinoma, PDTCs, and ATCs, PTCs have been shown to contain significantly higher numbers of DCs in surgical specimens.[6,31,36,44,45,50–56] In addition, DC density correlates with the degree of associated lymphocytic infiltration, both in tumoral tissue and in areas of thyroiditis.[45,53,56] DCs in PTC are mainly characterized by an immature phenotype (CD1a+) (**Fig. 1A, B**). Two early studies showed that PTC patients with a dense S100+ DC infiltrate in the tumor had a more favorable prognosis, irrespective of other morphologic and clinical features.[6,56] A relationship between the extent of DC infiltrates and the prognosis of PTC was not confirmed, however, in other subsequent studies.[45,53] PDTCs and ATCs were characterized by markedly reduced DC tumor infiltrates compared with PTC.[53]

MAST CELLS

MCs are bone marrow-derived immune cells that migrate into tissues where they are widely distributed throughout and mature depending on microenvironmental conditions.[11,57,58] MCs are characterized by cytoplasmic secretory granules that vary considerably in their cytokine and proteolytic enzyme content.[11] MCs are one of the most versatile cells in the body, owing to their ubiquitous location and the abundance of biologically active molecules that they produce, including pro- and antitumorigenic factors.[11,57] Although best known for their role in allergy and anaphylaxis, MCs are present in many tumors, affecting angiogenesis, tumor invasion of the extracellular matrix through the release of cytokines and proteases, and metastasis.[57–59] The protumorigenic role of MCs in cancer is supported by the observation that cancer growth is greatly reduced in MC-deficient mice and increased density, in human carcinomas, correlates with a dismal prognosis.[58,59] Conversely, MCs may also induce tumor cell apoptosis or stimulate T-cell–mediated cytotoxicity.

MAST CELLS IN NORMAL THYROID AND IN PAPILLARY THYROID CARCINOMA

In the normal thyroid gland, MCs are rare or absent, akin to DCs. Melillo and colleagues[58] have shown using immunohistochemistry with tryptase

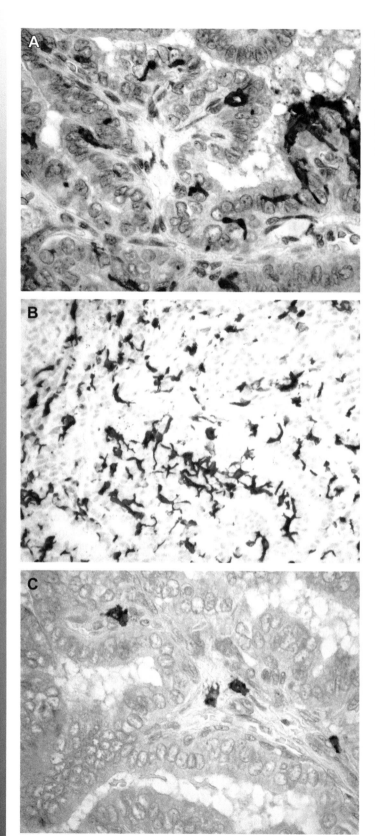

Fig. 1. CD1a immunostain reveals numerous DCs with cytoplasmic extensions in PTC on histology (*A*, CD1a immunostain, magnification ×400; *B*, CD1a immunostain, magnification ×100) and on cytology (*E*, CD1a immunostain, magnification ×200). CD117 immunostain reveals several MCs in PTC (*C*, CD117 immunostain, magnification ×400).

Fig. 1. (*continued*). Warthinlike variant of PTC: the tumor cells have an oncocytic appearance, and the stroma contains numerous lymphocytes reminiscent of a Warthin tumor of the salivary gland (*D*, Hematoxylin-eosin stain, magnification ×100). ATC (*F*, Hematoxylin-eosin stain, magnification ×400) contains numerous TAMs that are positive on CD68 immunostain (*G*, CD68 immunostain, magnification ×200; *H*, CD68 immunostain, magnification ×400). TAMs are difficult to recognize on hematoxylineosin stain (*E*) and show a peculiar morphology with cytoplasmic extension between tumor cells (*H*).

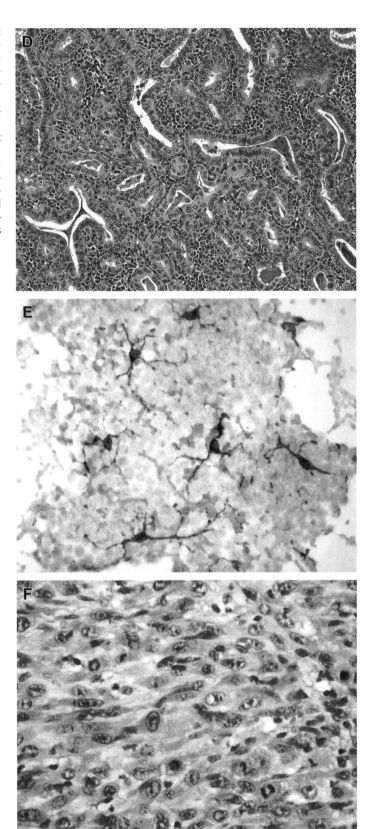

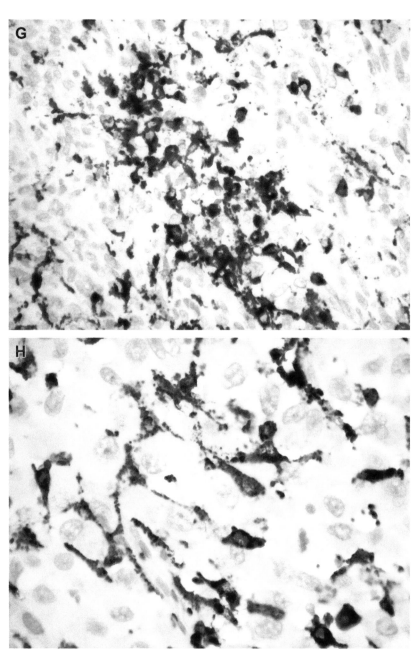

Fig. 1. (continued). ATC (F) contains numerous TAMs that are positive on CD68 immunostain (G, H). TAMs are difficult to recognize on hematoxyli-neosin stain (E) and show a peculiar morphology with cytoplasmic extension between tumor cells (H).

that MC density was higher in 95% of PTCs than in control tissue (see Fig. 1C). Thus, the presence of MC infiltrate distinguished normal thyroid tissue from PTC (P = .0001). Moreover, the extent of MC infiltration in PTCs was found positively correlated with capsule invasion, extrathyroidal extension, and poor prognosis. Using chemoattraction assays, Melillo and colleagues[58] showed that PTCs attract MCs through the release of VEGF-A. Once recruited, MCs may promote proliferation, survival, and invasive ability of cancer cells through MC-derived mediators, including histamine and chemokines, such as chemokine (C-X-C motif) ligand (CXCL) 1 and CXCL10.[50,58] Therefore, MCs seem to contribute to PTC growth and invasiveness.

TUMOR-INFILTRATING MACROPHAGES

Akin to DCs and MCs, macrophages also differentiate from bone marrow progenitors and are mobilized from the bone marrow into the periphery, where they differentiate into monocytes and, after homing into a tissue, mature into macrophages or histiocytes. Macrophage infiltration of tumors is also controlled by cytokines, growth factors, and enzymes secreted by the primary tumor.[60] The role of macrophages in tumor growth and development is complex, but TAMs are generally considered protumorigenic and associated with poor prognosis.[12,29,61,62] Low macrophage number has been correlated with inhibition of tumor growth and metastasis in different animal models.[30] There are some exceptions, however, with a high density of TAMs correlating with increased survival in some tumors, including pancreatic carcinoma.[62] TAMs secrete several chemokines and growth factors that produce paracrine effects on tumor cells, supporting tumor progression; TAM-derived chemokines may directly enhance tumor cell growth and may indirectly influence thyroid cancer cell expression of chemokine receptors, such as CXCR4,[26] that are important for tumor spread and metastasis.[63] Furthermore, secretion of matrix metalloproteases by TAMs can remodel the extracellular matrix, thus allowing tumor cell mobility, migration, and invasion at both local and distant sites. TAMs are classified in 2 major phenotypes: the classically activated type M1 phenotype and the alternative activated type M2 phenotype.[62] M1 macrophages show tumor-suppressive functions and are capable of killing microorganisms or tumor cells. In contrast, M2 macrophages (CD163+) have tumor-promoting functions and have important roles in angiogenesis, lymphangiogenesis, matrix remodeling, and tumor metastasis. TAMs typically have an M2 phenotype and a high density of M2 macrophages has been associated with more aggressive behavior and poor outcome in many malignant tumors.[12,30,61]

TUMOR-ASSOCIATED MACROPHAGES IN THE THYROID GLAND AND IN THYROID CANCER

The overall density of TAMs was shown significantly higher in PTC compared with goiter and FA.[56,64] In an early study, Fiumara and colleagues[56] found using immunohistochemistry with CD68 that TAMs were present in approximately 70% of PTCs (n = 121). Phagocytosis of neoplastic cells by macrophages, suggesting M1 phenotype and activity, was observed in approximately 15% of PTCs, and none of these tumors metastasized.[6] Moreover, neoplastic cell phagocytosis was strongly associated with the presence of DC and lymphocytic infiltration. The role of TAMs in thyroid cancer was subsequently studied by other investigators who found that a high density of TAMs positively correlates with tumor invasion, lymph node metastasis and TNM stage, and decreased cancer-related survival in PTC.[12] Furthermore, TAM infiltration was significantly increased in PDTCs and ATCs compared with PTCs.[12,29,64] More specifically, an increased density of M2 TAMs was associated with higher tumor grade and with decreased survival.[12,64] In contrast, Fiumara and colleagues[56] did not observe an association between the presence of TAMs and extrathyroidal extension, lymph node or distant metastases in PTC. Their study was limited, however, to patients with favorable outcomes, and they did not characterize the phenotype (M1 vs M2) of TAMs. Taken together, these data support the role of TAMs, especially of M2 type, as tumor-promoting and tumor-supporting cells in thyroid cancer.[12,50,64]

CHRONIC LYMPHOCYTIC THYROIDITIS AND THYROID CARCINOMA

The epidemiologic association of CLT and thyroid cancer, mostly PTC, is reported with variable frequency in the literature, ranging from no evidence of association to a 38% association.[2,3,45] The lymphocytic infiltration within PTC was found to correlate with the severity of thyroiditis in the nontumorous tissue, suggesting that immunologic mechanisms play a role in their pathogenesis.[4] In support of this, the Warthin-like variant of PTC, which is composed predominantly of papillae filled with a dense lymphoplasmacytic infiltrate and lined by oncocytic cells, is frequently associated with CLT (see Fig. 1D).

Numerous studies indicate that PTC with lymphocytic infiltrates in a background of CLT is associated with a less extensive disease at diagnosis and improved disease-free survival.[56,65] French and colleagues[16] found, however, that in the absence of CLT, patients with tumor-infiltrating lymphocytes in PTC exhibited higher disease stage and increased incidence of invasion and lymph node metastasis compared with patients without lymphocytes.

T LYMPHOCYTES

T lymphocytes (T cells) play a central role in the immune response against pathogens and tumors. Tumor-infiltrating T cells are generally a predictor of a positive clinical outcome in cancer.[66] Subset analyses revealed, however, that although infiltration by cytotoxic (CD8+) T cells is a positive prognostic indicator, infiltration by Tregs is a negative prognostic indicator in several malignancies.[15,16,38] Previous studies have shown that increased numbers of infiltrating CD4$^+$ and CD8$^+$ effector T lymphocytes are correlated with lower-stage disease and longer disease-free survival in PTC patients.[67] T-helper (CD4$^+$) and cytotoxic (CD8$^+$) lymphocytes are directly involved in cell-mediated tumor destruction whereas Tregs may contribute to immune system evasion, acting as immunosuppressants.

REGULATORY T CELLS

Tregs inhibit T-cell proliferation and maintain tolerance to self-antigens by the secretion of inhibitory cytokines and/or contact-mediated inhibition.[15,16,68–71] There is increasing evidence that Tregs also function in cancer immune evasion. Increased Tregs, whether in the primary tumor, draining lymph nodes, or blood, have been associated with poor prognosis in many cancers.[16,68–71] Tregs are CD4$^+$CD25$^+$ T cells that specifically express forkhead box P3 (FoxP3), a transcription factor that is essential for the development and function of these cells. In the thyroid, 3 studies by 2 groups found that the presence of CD4$^+$CD25$^+$FoxP3$^+$ Tregs in PTC correlated with more aggressive disease, more advanced stage, and more lymph node metastasis.[15,16,70] Expression of FoxP3 has also been reported on tumor cells and seems associated with a negative prognosis in several cancers, including PTC.[16,63,69,70]

NATURAL KILLER CELLS

NK cells recognize and destroy invading pathogens and are, therefore, important effector cells of innate immunity. They are a minor subset of lymphocytes without specific B- or T-cell antigens.[72] The NK-cell subsets exhibit important differences in their cytotoxic potential, capacity for cytokine production, and response to cytokine activation. The major subset of NK cells (CD56 dim) is cytotoxic, whereas a minor subset (CD56 bright) plays an immunoregulatory role. Immunoregulatory NK cells produce several cytokines, including interferon γ, tumor necrosis factor (TNF)-α, and granulocyte-macrophage colony-stimulating factor (GM-CSF), whereas cytotoxic NK cells produce proteases (eg, granzymes and perforin) that facilitate apoptosis. The role of NK cells has been widely studied in several malignancies, although only recently in thyroid cancer. Gogali and colleagues[72] found increased NK cells (mainly CD56 bright subtype) in thyroid tissue of patients with PTC compared with those with nodular goiter. Furthermore, they found a negative correlation between NK infiltration in PTC tumor tissue and disease stage, together with an increase in the ratio between CD56 dim and CD56 bright NK cells with disease stage.[15,72]

THE ROLE OF CYTOKINES/CHEMOKINES IN THYROID CANCER

Cancer cells attract inflammatory cells through the release of many chemokines. Chemokines, a subgroup of cytokines, are subdivided into 4 subfamilies, namely CXC, CC, C, and CX3C, based on the arrangement of 4 conserved cysteine residues within the protein. They induce cell migration and activation by binding to specific G protein–coupled cell-surface receptors on target cells (CCRs). Cytokines and chemokines that play a role in thyroid cancer are shown in **Table 1**. Tumor-derived cell lines from WDTCs and ATCs have been shown to secrete several cytokines/chemokines, including CXCL1, granulocyte colony-stimulating factor, GM-CSF, IL-1a, IL-6, IL-8, monocyte chemotactic protein-1 (MCP-1), and TNF-α.[6,20–26] The role of cytokines/chemokines in thyroid cancer has been studied mostly in PTC. Oncoproteins typically expressed in PTCs, such as RET/PTC, RAS, and BRAF, trigger a proinflammatory program in tumor cells by upregulation of several chemokines.[20–26] For example, RET/PTC induces the expression of oncogenes involved in inflammation and tumor invasion, including chemokines (chemokine [C-C motif] ligand [CCL] 2, CCL20, CXCL8, and CXCL12), chemokine receptor CXCR4, and cytokines (IL-1B, colony-stimulating factor 1, and GM-CSF).[22,24] Thyrocytes engineered to express RET/PTC3 have also been shown to produce high amounts of MCP-1, GM-CSF, CXCL10, and IL-6.[24] Muzza and colleagues[20] demonstrated that the genes encoding chemokines CCL20, CXCL8, and the adhesion molecule L-selectin were overexpressed in PTC compared with normal thyroid, regardless of RET/PTC or BRAF status, and suggested that CXCL8 and CCL20 could be associated with tumor-related inflammation. PTC cells are also characterized by overexpression of Met protein, the receptor for hepatocyte growth factor (HGF), in 95% of cases.[6] It has been demonstrated that HGF/Met interaction is biologically active in PTC, leading to the release of chemokines, such as macrophage inflammatory protein (MIP)-1α (CCL20), MIP-1β and MIP-3α.[6] In contrast, FTC, which does not overexpress Met protein, shows no significant TAICs.[6] Among the many cytokines produced by PTC, VEGF-A attracts MCs,[58] whereas CCL2 attracts macrophages/monocytes.[60] Finally, MIP-3α, MIP-1β, MIP-3α, IL-1-α, and TNF-α, which are also expressed strongly in a majority of PTC but weakly in FTC,[36,54] attract DCs.[6,20,22]

Table 1
Selected cytokines and chemokines that play major roles in thyroid carcinoma

	Other Name	Receptor(s)	Main Effects on Tumor Cells	Main Effects on Tumor-Associated Inflammatory Cells	References
Chemokines					
CCL2	MCP-1	CCR2	Pro- or antitumorigenic depending on concentration	Attraction of macrophages, MCs, and immature DCs. M2 macrophages polarization	5,22,38
CXCL1	GROα	CXCR2	Proliferation and invasion	Attraction of neutrophils	25,38,58
CXCL8	IL-8	CXCR1, CXCR2	Proliferation, invasion, and metastasis	Attraction of leukocytes	38
CXCL10	IP-10	CXCR3	Proliferation and invasion	Attraction of macrophages, T cells, NK cells, and DCs	25,38,58
CXCL12	SDF-1	CXCR4, CXCR7	Proliferation and metastasis	Accumulation of Tregs and pDCs	5,22,26,38,63
CCL3	MIP-1α	CCR1		Attraction of DCs	6
CCL4	MIP-1β	CCR1, CCR5		Attraction of DCs	6
CCL20	MIP-3α	CCR6	Migration	Attraction of macrophages and immature DCs	6,17,22,34,37
Cytokines					
IL-1α/IL-1β		IL1-RI	Growth inhibition	DC maturation	22,23
IL-6	Interferon-β2	IL6R (CD126)	Proliferation	Inhibition of DC differentiation and maturation. M2 macrophages polarization	5,17,38
CSF-1	M-CSF	CSF1R (CD115)		Controls the production, differentiation, and function of macrophages	38
GM-CSF		GM-CSFR (CD116)		Accumulation of immature DCs with inhibitory functions	17
VEGF-A		VEGFR1, VEGFR2	Proliferation, migration, and survival (autocrine)	Attraction of MCs, DCs and macrophages. Inhibits functionnal maturation of DCs	11,46
TNF-α	Cachexin	TNFR1, TNFR2	Proliferation, migration, and resistance to drugs	Accumulation of immature DCs with inhibitory functions	23
TGF-β		TGF-β receptors	Invasion, repression of sodium/iodide transporter	Converts effector T cells to Tregs	38
HGF		c-Met receptor	Proliferation and invasion	Suppression of Ag-presenting capacity of DCs	6,38

Abbreviations: IP-10, interferon gamma-induced protein 10; M-CSF, macrophage colony-stimulating factor; SDF-1, stromal cell–derived factor 1.

TUMOR-ASSOCIATED INFLAMMATORY CELLS IN PAPILLARY THYROID CARCINOMA VARIANTS

Some PTC variants are associated with a better prognosis than classical PTC (eg, follicular variant of PTC [FVPTC]), whereas others are associated with more aggressive behavior, with a propensity for lymph node metastasis and/or reduced sensitivity to radioiodine treatment (eg, diffuse sclerosing variant of PTC [DSVPTC] and tall cell, columnar cell, and hobnail variants). Scarce data are available on TAICs in other variants of PTC and are reviewed later.

FOLLICULAR VARIANT OF PAPILLARY THYROID CARCINOMA

FVPTC is the second most common form of PTC, after classical type, and is associated with an excellent prognosis, especially in cases lacking vascular and/or capsular invasion.[73] This variant is composed entirely of follicles lined by cells with nuclear features of PTC, either focally or throughout the tumor, with crowding, nuclear clearing, membrane irregularities, and grooves. Most FVPTCs are encapsulated, and the diagnosis of this variant has marked interobserver variability, even among expert thyroid pathologists.[73] FVPTC is a hybrid tumor, with morphologic, molecular, biological, and clinical features bridging FA, minimally invasive FTC, and classical PTC. Proietti and colleagues[50] assessed the presence of TAICs, including mature and immature DCs, MCs, and TAMs in consecutive FVPTCs (n = 91) and FAs (n = 44). They observed significantly greater numbers of intralesional and perilesional CD1a+ DCs in FVPTCs compared with FAs (P = .0001). Intralesional and perilesional CD1a+ DCs were present, however, in only 46% and 21% of FVPTCs, respectively, and in 3% of FAs.[50] This contrasts with the higher reported rates of DCs in classical PTC.[31,36,44,45,51,52,54,55] The investigators also assessed the presence of mature DCs (DC-LAMP+), but no differences were observed between FVPTCs and FAs.[50] The FVPTCs contained no or sparse lymphocyte infiltrates together with low amount of DCs. The lower inflammatory response seen in FVPTC compared with classical PTC may be related to several factors, including a lower expression of tumor antigens and/or detection of tumor antigens by DCs, a lower amount of cytokine/chemokine production and/or secretion that may be related in part to the lower prevalence of BRAF or RET/PTC alterations in FVPTC, and finally tumor encapsulation, which is a common feature of FVPTCs. In support of these hypotheses, a higher amount of MCs was found in the peritumoral compartment of nonencapsulated FVPTCs, which are known to harbor BRAF mutations more commonly than encapsulated FVPTCs. More controversially, this may also indicate absence of malignancy in a subset of this group prone to subjective diagnosis.

DIFFUSE SCLEROSING VARIANT OF PAPILLARY THYROID CARCINOMA

The diffuse sclerosing variant of PTC (DSVPTC) is associated with a more aggressive biological behavior than classical PTC. It is characterized by stromal fibrosis, dense lymphocytic infiltrates, and extensive lymphatic invasion with lymph node metastasis at the time of diagnosis in most cases. Recently, Chang and colleagues[74] found a strong correlation between increased M2 TAMs and lymphatic invasion in the DSVPTC. In their study, the lymphatic tumor emboli were closely admixed with TAMs and contained a relatively higher density of TAMs than stroma and PTC areas. In addition, the number of M2 TAMs correlated with the size of the tumor emboli, with older patients and larger tumor size.[74] The investigators also showed that PTC tumor cells in tumor emboli, but not in solid tumor areas, expressed decoy receptor 3 (DcR3), and that DcR3 expression was positively associated with M2 differentiation, lymphatic invasion, and size of emboli.[74] DcR3 can actually modulate macrophage differentiation in TAMs toward the M2 phenotype. That lymphatic emboli in DSVPTC are a heterogeneous population consisting of tumor cells and mostly M2 TAMs suggests that TAMs play an important role in the process of lymphatic invasion in DSVPTC.[74]

TUMOR-ASSOCIATED INFLAMMATORY CELLS IN FINE-NEEDLE ASPIRATION BIOPSIES OF PAPILLARY THYROID CARCINOMA

Because fine-needle aspiration biopsy (FNAB) is the leading method for the initial evaluation of a thyroid nodule and for the diagnosis of PTC, the presence of TAICs in thyroid FNAB may be helpful for diagnostic purposes in cases with indeterminate cytology. Moreover, the identification of cytomorphologic factors or molecular factors (eg, BRAF V600E mutation) predicting lymph node metastasis is clinically important for determining the appropriate treatment due to the high rate of lymph node involvement by PTC at the time of diagnosis. Therefore, the identification of TAICs, such as M2-macrophages, which have been positively associated with lymph node metastasis,[74] in FNABs of PTC may be important for prognostic and therapeutic purposes.[64] No study investigating this question specifically has been published, however. Recently, the authors have shown by immunocytochemistry that immature (CD1a[+]) DCs can also be identified in cytologic specimens from most PTC (97%) (see Fig. 1E), correlating with histology (see Fig. 1A, B), and significantly more numerous than in benign thyroid.[31] DCs can be found in close association with PTC cells where they exhibit long dendritic cytoplasmic extensions in-between and around tumor cells (see Fig. 1E). The authors suggest that the increased presence of CD1a[+] DCs in PTC may be a useful diagnostic marker in thyroid FNAB but did not find, however, any association between the amount of DCs in PTC and other clinicopathological parameters in this small series. The authors found similar results with MCs in thyroid FNAB from PTC (Pusztaszeri MP, unpublished data, 2013), supporting the results of the studies discussed previously on surgical resection specimens of PTC. Further investigation of TAICs in cytologic material is warranted to assess for diagnostic/prognostic utility.

TUMOR-ASSOCIATED INFLAMMATORY CELLS IN POORLY DIFFERENTIATED THYROID CARCINOMAS AND ANAPLASTIC THYROID CARCINOMAS

Although ATC represents less than 5% of all thyroid cancer, it is one of the most aggressive malignancies in humans, with most patients dying within a year of diagnosis. PDTC is intermediate between WDTC and ATC in terms of its morphology, molecular alterations, biological behavior, and prognosis.

PDTCs and ATCs are both characterized by strongly reduced lymphocyte and DC infiltrates compared with PTC, suggesting that these cells may play a protective role in thyroid cancer.[53] In contrast, Ryder and colleagues[12] found that the amount of TAMs was higher in PDTCs and ATCs than in WDTCs. Moreover, increased TAMs in PDTCs were associated with capsular invasion, extrathyroidal extension, and decreased cancer-related survival compared with PDTCs with a low density of TAMs.[12] ATC is characterized by a very dense network of TAMs, representing more than 50% of nucleated cells (see Fig. 1F–H).[29] These cells have a peculiar morphology, referred to as "ramified TAM" (RTAM) by Caillou and colleagues[29] and form an interconnected network in close contact with cancer cells, other TAMs, and blood vessels.[29] Electron microscopy revealed that TAMs in ATC display long, thin cytoplasmic processes extending up to 150 μm from the cell

body.[29] These cytoplasmic processes are often irregular and ramified conferring a microglial appearance (see Fig. 1H), appearing strikingly similar to DCs in PTC (see Fig. 1A, B). The morphology of RTAM contrasts with M1 macrophages, which are more rounded without major cytoplasmic extensions. Caillou and colleagues[29] suggested that these peculiar cytoplasmic extensions of RTAM may permit cross-talk and molecular transfers between RTAM and cancer cells and that the interconnected RTAM network in ATC may also play a vessel-like role in supplying nutrients from the blood to cancer cells. Taken together, these data also support the concept that TAMs may favor malignant progression in thyroid, with a supportive role in ATCs. Furthermore, some TAM-associated cytokines, such as TNF-α, may induce resistance to drugs.[12]

TAMs in ATCs may have potential diagnostic and therapeutic applications. On imaging, PDTC and ATC typically display an intense uptake of fludeoxyglucose F 18 (18FDG) on PET but do not uptake iodine on scintigraphy due to loss of the sodium-iodine symporter (NIS) related to tumor dedifferentiation.[75] In contrast, WDTCs whose tumor cells express NIS, enabling them to trap iodine, show a reverse pattern on imaging (flip-flop phenomenon).[75] Moreover, a strong positive correlation has been found between the presence of the glucose transporter glucose transporter 1 (GLUT-1) and 18FDG uptake in thyroid tumors.[76] GLUT-1 expression also correlates with the degree of differentiation of thyroid tumors, more intensely expressed in ATCs than in WDTCs.[77] Caillou and colleagues[29] showed, however, that although a majority of cancer cells in ATCs were negative for GLUT-1, only blood vessels and a subset of RTAM were positive for GLUT-1. This supports the notion that glucose uptake from the blood takes place mainly in RTAM rather than in cancer cells.[29] Therefore, these data suggest that the high fludeoxyglucose uptake in ATCs could be mostly related to the high number of TAMs and that the RTAM network plays a major role for the glucose metabolism in ATCs.[29]

A better understanding of the role of TAM in thyroid cancer is crucial for therapeutic development. Vigorous efforts are underway to develop novel therapies for thyroid cancer, specifically interfering with signaling pathways activated by mutated oncoproteins (targeted therapies) or increasing tumor sensitivity to radioactive iodine in resistant tumors, such as PDTCs and ATCs. These therapeutic approaches also to need take into account, however, the important tumor supportive role of TAM, especially in poorly differentiated tumors, for therapeutic efficacy.

SUMMARY

The immune system is integral in the evolution of certain thyroid cancers where it plays a complex role. This is reflected by the diversity of TAIC phenotypes, including state of activation and cytokine production, both pro- and antitumorigenic. The assessment of immune cells and immune response in thyroid cancer may be relevant to its diagnosis, prognosis, and management. Although current therapies, primarily surgery, are effective for most patients with thyroid cancer, a significant number of patients with PTC develop recurrences that may be resistant to conventional treatment. For this subset of patients, as well as for patients with more aggressive thyroid malignancies, certain features of the complex tumor-immune system interaction suggest that key TAIC subsets may have a role as novel cancer cell–oriented targeted therapies.

REFERENCES

1. Virchow R. Die Krankhaften Geschwulste. Verlag von August Hirschwald; Berlin: 1863. Aetologie der neoplastichen Geschwulste/Pathogenie der neoplastischen Geschwulste. p. 57–101.
2. Di Pasquale M, Rothstein JL, Palazzo JP. Pathologic features of Hashimoto's-associated papillary thyroid carcinomas. Hum Pathol 2001;32: 24–30.
3. Ott RA, McCall AR, McHenry C, et al. The incidence of thyroid carcinoma in Hashimoto's thyroiditis. Am Surg 1987;53:442–5.
4. Okayasu I, Fujiwara M, Hara Y, et al. Association of chronic lymphocytic thyroiditis and thyroid papillary carcinoma. A study of surgical cases among Japanese, and white and African Americans. Cancer 1995;76:2312–8.
5. Germano G, Allavena P, Mantovani A. Cytokines as a key component of cancer-related inflammation. Cytokine 2008;43:374–9.
6. Scarpino S, Stoppacciaro A, Ballerini F, et al. Papillary carcinoma of the thyroid: hepatocyte growth factor (HGF) stimulates tumor cells to release chemokines active in recruiting dendritic cells. Am J Pathol 2000;156:831–7.
7. Hanahan D, Weinberg RA. Hallmarks of cancer: the next generation. Cell 2011;144:646–74.
8. Penn I. Depressed immunity and the development of cancer. Cancer Detect Prev 1994;18:241–52.
9. Rothwell PM, Price JF, Fowkes FG, et al. Short-term effects of daily aspirin on cancer incidence, mortality, and non-vascular death: analysis of the time course of risks and benefits in 51 randomised controlled trials. Lancet 2012;379: 1602–12.
10. Hart DN. Dendritic cells: unique leukocyte populations which control the primary immune response. Blood 1997;90:3245–87.
11. Theoharides TC, Conti P. Mast cells: the Jekyll and Hyde of tumor growth. Trends Immunol 2004;25: 235–41.
12. Ryder M, Ghossein RA, Ricarte-Filho JC, et al. Increased density of tumor-associated macrophages is associated with decreased survival in advanced thyroid cancer. Endocr Relat Cancer 2008;15:1069–74.
13. Karthaus N, Torensma R, Tel J. Deciphering the message broadcast by tumor-infiltrating dendritic cells. Am J Pathol 2012;181:733–42.
14. Mantovani A, Schioppa T, Porta C, et al. Role of tumor-associated macrophages in tumor progression and invasion. Cancer Metastasis Rev 2006; 25:315–22.
15. Gogali F, Paterakis G, Rassidakis GZ, et al. Phenotypical analysis of lymphocytes with suppressive and regulatory properties (Tregs) and NK cells in the papillary carcinoma of thyroid. J Clin Endocrinol Metab 2012;97:1474–82.
16. French JD, Weber ZJ, Fretwell DL, et al. Tumor-associated lymphocytes and increased FoxP3+ regulatory T cell frequency correlate with more aggressive papillary thyroid cancer. J Clin Endocrinol Metab 2010;95:2325–33.
17. Pinzon-Charry A, Maxwell T, Lopez JA. Dendritic cell dysfunction in cancer: a mechanism for immunosuppression. Immunol Cell Biol 2005;83:451–61.
18. Vicari AP, Caux C, Trinchieri G. Tumour escape from immune surveillance through dendritic cell inactivation. Semin Cancer Biol 2002;12:33–42.
19. Kimura ET, Nikiforova MN, Zhu Z, et al. High prevalence of BRAF mutations in thyroid cancer: genetic evidence for constitutive activation of the RET/PTC-RAS-BRAF signaling pathway in papillary thyroid carcinoma. Cancer Res 2003;63:1454–7.
20. Muzza M, Degl'Innocenti D, Colombo C, et al. The tight relationship between papillary thyroid cancer, autoimmunity and inflammation: clinical and molecular studies. Clin Endocrinol (Oxf) 2010;72:702–8.
21. Guarino V, Castellone MD, Avilla E, et al. Thyroid cancer and inflammation. Mol Cell Endocrinol 2010;321:94–102.
22. Borrello MG, Alberti L, Fischer A, et al. Induction of a proinflammatory program in normal human thyrocytes by the RET/PTC1 oncogene. Proc Natl Acad Sci U S A 2005;102:14825–30.
23. Russel JP, Shinohara S, Melillo RM, et al. Tyrosine kinase oncoprotein, RET/PTC3, induces the secretion of myeloid growth and chemotactic factors. Oncogene 2003;22:4569–77.
24. Puxeddu E, Knauf JA, Sartor MA, et al. RET/PTC induced gene expression in thyroid PCCL3 cells reveals early activation of genes involved in

regulation of the immune response. Endocr Relat Cancer 2005;12:319–34.

25. Melillo RM, Castellone MD, Guarino V, et al. The RET/PTC-RAS-BRAF linear signaling cascade mediates the motile and mitogenic phenotype of thyroid cancer cells. J Clin Invest 2005;115:1068–81.

26. Castellone MD, Guarino V, De Falco V, et al. Functional expression of the CXCR4 chemokine receptor is induced by RET/PTC oncogenes and is a common event in human papillary thyroid carcinomas. Oncogene 2004;23:5958–67.

27. Zong YS, Zhang CQ, Zhang F, et al. Infiltrating lymphocytes and accessory cells in nasopharyngeal carcinoma. Jpn J Cancer Res 1993;84:900–5.

28. Hadrup SR, Braendstrup O, Jacobsen GK, et al. Tumor infiltrating lymphocytes in semi-noma lesions comprise clonally expanded cytotoxic T cells. Int J Cancer 2006;119:831–8.

29. Caillou B, Talbot M, Weyemi U, et al. Tumor-associated macrophages (TAMs) form an interconnected cellular supportive network in anaplastic thyroid carcinoma. PLoS One 2011;6:e22567.

30. Solinas G, Germano G, Mantovani A, et al. Tumor-associated macrophages (TAM) as major players of the cancer-related inflammation. J Leukoc Biol 2009;86:1065–73.

31. Pusztaszeri MP, Sadow PM, Faquin WC. Association of CD1a-positive dendritic cells with papillary thyroid carcinoma in thyroid fine-needle aspirations: a cytologic and immunocytochemical evaluation. Cancer Cytopathol 2013;121:206–13.

32. Finak G, Bertos N, Pepin F, et al. Stromal gene expression predicts clinical outcome in breast cancer. Nat Med 2008;14:518–27.

33. Cella M, Sallusto F, Lanzavecchia A. Origin, maturation and antigen presenting function of dendritic cells. Curr Opin Immunol 1997;9:10–6.

34. Bell D, Chomarat P, Broyles D, et al. In breast carcinoma tissue, immature dendritic cells reside within the tumor, whereas mature dendritic cells are located in peritumoral areas. J Exp Med 1999;190:1417–26.

35. Bancherau J, Steinman RM. Dendritic cells and control of immunity. Nature 1998;392:245–52.

36. Tsuge K, Takeda H, Kawada S, et al. Characterization of dendritic cells in differentiated thyroid cancer. J Pathol 2005;205:565–76.

37. Greaves DR, Wang W, Dairaghi DJ, et al. CCR6, a CC chemokine receptor that interacts with macrophage inflammatory protein 3 alpha and is highly expressed in human dendritic cells. J Exp Med 1997;186:837–44.

38. Talmadge JE, Donkor M, Scholar E. Inflammatory cell infiltration of tumors: Jekyll or Hyde. Cancer Metastasis Rev 2007;26:373–400.

39. Leskela S, Rodríguez-Muñoz A, de la Fuente H, et al. Plasmacytoid dendritic cells in patients with autoimmune thyroid disease. J Clin Endocrinol Metab 2013;98:2822–33.

40. Yu H, Huang X, Liu X, et al. Regulatory T cells and plasmacytoid dendritic cells contribute to the immune escape of papillary thyroid cancer coexisting with multinodular non-toxic goiter. Endocrine 2013;44:172–81.

41. Ma Y, Shurin GV, Peiyuan Z, et al. Dendritic cells in the cancer microenvironment. J Cancer 2013;4:36–44.

42. Hanke N, Alizadeh D, Katsanis E, et al. Dendritic cell tumor killing activity and its potential applications in cancer immunotherapy. Crit Rev Immunol 2013;33:1–21.

43. Sandel MH, Dadabayev AR, Menon AG, et al. Prognostic value of tumor-infiltrating dendritic cells in colorectal cancer: role of maturation status and intratumoral localization. Clin Cancer Res 2005;11:2576–82.

44. Schröder S, Schwarz W, Rehpenning W, et al. Dendritic/Langerhans cells and prognosis in patients with papillary thyroid carcinomas. Immunocytochemical study of 106 thyroid neoplasms correlated to follow-up data. Am J Clin Pathol 1988;89:295–300.

45. Hilly O, Koren R, Raz R, et al. The role of s100-positive dendritic cells in the prognosis of papillary thyroid carcinoma. Am J Clin Pathol 2013;139:87–92.

46. Gabrilovich D. Mechanisms and functional significance of tumour induced dendritic cell defects. Nat Rev Immunol 2004;4:941–52.

47. Enk AH, Jonuleit H, Saloga J, et al. Dendritic cells as mediators of tumor-induced tolerance in metastatic melanoma. Int J Cancer 1997;73:309–16.

48. Yamakawa M, Kato H, Takagi S, et al. Dendritic cells in various human thyroid diseases. In Vivo 1993;7:249–56.

49. Kabel PJ, Voorbij HA, De Haan M, et al. Intrathyroidal dendritic cells. Clin Endocrinol Metab 1988;66:199–207.

50. Proietti A, Ugolini C, Melillo RM, et al. Higher intratumoral expression of CD1a, tryptase, and CD68 in a follicular variant of papillary thyroid carcinoma compared to adenomas: correlation with clinical and pathological parameters. Thyroid 2011;21:1209–15.

51. McLaren KM, Cossar DW. The immunohistochemical localization of S100 in the diagnosis of papillary carcinoma of the thyroid. Hum Pathol 1996;27:633–6.

52. Xu W, Li X, Chen S, et al. Expression and distribution of S-100, CD83 and apoptosis-related proteins (Fas, FasL and Bcl-2) in tissues of thyroid carcinoma. Eur J Histochem 2008;52:153–62.

53. Ugolini C, Basolo F, Proietti A, et al. Lymphocyte and immature dendritic cell infiltrates in differentiated,

poorly differentiated, and undifferentiated thyroid carcinoma. Thyroid 2007;17:389–93.

54. Yamakawa M, Yamada K, Orui H, et al. Immunohistochemical analysis of dendritic/Langerhans cells in thyroid carcinomas. Anal Cell Pathol 1995;8:331–43.

55. Batistatou A, Zolota V, Scopa CD. S-100 protein+ dendritic cells and CD34+ dendritic interstitial cells in thyroid lesions. Endocr Pathol 2002;13:111–5.

56. Fiumara A, Belfiore A, Russo G, et al. In situ evidence of neoplastic cell phagocytosis by macrophages in papillary thyroid cancer. J Clin Endocrinol Metab 1997;82:1615–20.

57. Khazaie K, Blatner NR, Khan MW, et al. The significant role of mast cells in cancer. Cancer Metastasis Rev 2011;30:45–60.

58. Melillo RM, Guarino V, Avilla E, et al. Mast cells have a protumorigenic role in human thyroid cancer. Oncogene 2010;29:6203–15.

59. Takanami I, Takeuchi K, Naruke M. Mast cell density is associated with angiogenesis and poor prognosis in pulmonary adenocarcinoma. Cancer 2000;88:2686–92.

60. Pollard JW. Trophic macrophages in development and disease. Nat Rev Immunol 2009;9:259–70.

61. Bingle L, Brown NJ, Lewis CE. The role of tumour-associated macrophages in tumour progression: implications for new anticancer therapies. J Pathol 2002;196:254–65.

62. Zhang QW, Liu L, Gong CY, et al. Prognostic significance of tumor-associated macrophages in solid tumor: a meta-analysis of the literature. PLoS One 2012;7:e50946.

63. Ugolini C, Elisei R, Proietti A, et al. FoxP3 expression in papillary thyroid carcinoma: a possible resistance biomarker to iodine 131 treatment. Thyroid 2014;24(2):339–46.

64. Qing W, Fang WY, Ye L, et al. Density of tumor-associated macrophages correlates with lymph node metastasis in papillary thyroid carcinoma. Thyroid 2012;22:905–10.

65. Matsubayashi S, Kawai K, Matsumoto Y, et al. The correlation between papillary thyroid carcinoma and lymphocytic infiltration in the thyroid gland. J Clin Endocrinol Metab 1995;80:3421–4.

66. Gooden MJ, de Bock GH, Leffers N, et al. The prognostic influence of tumour-infiltrating lymphocytes in cancer: a systematic review with meta-analysis. Br J Cancer 2011;105:93–103.

67. Gupta S, Patel A, Folstad A, et al. Infiltration of differentiated thyroid carcinoma by proliferating lymphocytes is associated with improved disease-free survival for children and young adults. J Clin Endocrinol Metab 2001;86:1346–54.

68. Fehérvari Z, Sakaguchi S. CD4+ Tregs and immune control. J Clin Invest 2004;114:1209–17.

69. Zhou G, Levitsky HI. Natural regulatory T cells and de novo-induced regulatory T cells contribute independently to tumour-specific tolerance. J Immunol 2007;178:2155–62.

70. French JD, Kotnis GR, Said S, et al. Programmed death-1+ T cells and regulatory T cells are enriched in tumor-involved lymph nodes and associated with aggressive features in papillary thyroid cancer. J Clin Endocrinol Metab 2012;97:E934–43.

71. Bates GJ, Fox SB, Han C, et al. Quantification of regulatory T cells enables the identification of high-risk breast cancer patients and those at risk of late relapse. J Clin Oncol 2006;24:5373–80.

72. Gogali F, Paterakis G, Rassidakis GZ, et al. CD3-CD16-CD56bright immunoregulatory NK Cells are increased in the tumor microenvironment and inversely correlate with advanced stages in patients with papillary thyroid cancer. Thyroid 2013;23(12):1561–8.

73. Liu J, Singh B, Tallini G, et al. Follicular variant of papillary thyroid carcinoma: a clinicopathologic study of a problematic entity. Cancer 2006;107:1255–64.

74. Chang WC, Chen JY, Lee CH, et al. Expression of decoy receptor 3 in diffuse sclerosing variant of papillary thyroid carcinoma: correlation with m2 macrophage differentiation and lymphatic invasion. Thyroid 2013;23:720–6.

75. Bongiovanni M, Paone G, Cariani L, et al. Cellular and molecular basis for thyroid cancer imaging in nuclear medicine. Clin Transl Imaging 2013;1:149–61.

76. Grabellus F, Nagarajah J, Bockisch A, et al. Glucose transporter 1 expression, tumor proliferation, and iodine/glucose uptake in thyroid cancer with emphasis on poorly differentiated thyroid carcinoma. Clin Nucl Med 2012;37:121–7.

77. Schönberger J, Rüschoff J, Grimm D, et al. Glucose transporter 1 gene expression is related to thyroid neoplasms with an unfavorable prognosis: an immunohistochemical study. Thyroid 2002;12:747–54.

Parathyroid
The Pathology of Hyperparathyroidism

Virginia A. LiVolsi, MD*, Kathleen T. Montone, MD,
Zubair N. Baloch, MD, PhD

KEYWORDS

- Hyperparathyroidism • Adenoma • Hyperplasia atypical adenoma • Carcinoma • Parafibromin

ABSTRACT

This review focuses on the pathologic entities associated with hyperparathyroidism in humans. A discussion of the lesions, their embryology, and pathologic features is included. Immunohistology, cytopathology, and a brief overview of molecular aspects of the lesion are included.

PARATHYROID PATHOLOGY

Surgical pathologists encounter parathyroid tissue in several different settings and hence must be cognizant of the role played by pathologists in these scenarios.

First, during intraoperative consultations, such as frozen section, a sample of a parathyroid may be identified by a pathologist in a portion of tissue thought to be a lymph node or a thyroid nodule by the operating surgeon performing a head and neck procedure. The parathyroid in this type of case is usually a normocellular gland with an equal ratio of fat to parenchymal cells. This straightforward situation is one of identification, and the literature suggests pathologists are excellent at performing this task.[1]

Second, a pathologist may be asked to diagnose an abnormal parathyroid, one that is associated with clinical hyperfunction and, therefore, hypercalcemia. In these cases, the pathologist should weigh the gland and after describing it transect it along its long axis and prepare a frozen section slide from a portion of the gland. Evaluation by hematoxylin-eosin (H&E) staining and a metachromatic stain is helpful to assess extracellular and intracellular fat and determine functional status of the gland. If the morphology is consistent with an adenoma (by presence of a rim of normal parathyroid and appropriate results on assessment of fat—discussed later), a definitive diagnosis may be rendered. Ideally, the surgeon also samples (by biopsy) another parathyroid gland for frozen section (to assess morphology and lipid content) to confirm uniglandular disease. In the event that 2 abnormal glands are identified, then additional samples of other glands may be needed to recognize 2 adenomas or multigland hyperplasia.[2,3]

In the third scenario, parathyroidectomy for hyperplasia (either primary, as in familial hyperparathyroidism or in multiple endocrine neoplasia [MEN] syndrome, or secondary to chronic renal failure or other rarer causes of secondary hyperparathyroidism) is performed. In these types of surgeries, the pathologist's role is one of identification of the tissue as abnormally cellular parathyroid. Only rarely is it necessary to consider or suggest a diagnosis of an autonomous parathyroid neoplasm is such patients.[3,4]

On rare occasions, a surgeon encounters unusual findings, such as invasive growth of a parathyroid lesion or enlarged lymph nodes, raising the suspicion of a carcinoma of the parathyroid. This is an exceptional event (discussed later). It is often a deferred diagnosis at the time of frozen section unless unequivocal invasion of soft tissue, esophageal wall, thyroid, or nodes is identified.[4,5]

Finally, in recent decades, newer imaging techniques and approaches to identified abnormalities

Disclosure: The authors declare they have nothing to disclose.
Department of Pathology and Laboratory Medicine, Perelman School of Medicine, University of Pennsylvania, 3400 Spruce Street, Philadelphia, PA 19104, USA
* Corresponding author.
E-mail address: linus@mail.med.upenn.edu

surgpath.theclinics.com

has led to newer "lesions," which may be encountered intraoperatively or on routine sections. These include postbiopsy fibrosis and trapping simulating invasion, postbiopsy infarction (total or partial) of an adenoma,[6] and, in rare instances, the spillage of abnormal parathyroid tissue leading to parathyromatosis.[7]

These various pathologic entities are discussed.

The diagnosis of hyperparathyroidism is easy because it is often asymptomatic or minimally symptomatic and is recognized on screening biochemical testing when elevation of serum calcium is noted. Because a great majority of patients with primary hyperparathyroidism have 1 abnormally functioning and enlarged gland, it seems simple that a surgical approach with removal of the offending gland would lead to cure. The role of the surgical pathologist is to identify the abnormal parathyroid and document its location and complete removal.[5,8,9]

The literature belies such a simplistic scenario. As those surgical pathologists who practiced before the middle 1990s can recall, the finding of a "parathyroid exploration" listed on an operating room schedule caused sadness and trepidation for the pathologists because they knew that many frozen sections would be performed in the search for the offending gland. Depending on the experience and expertise of the surgeon, as many as 10 to 20 individual frozen section samples (many fat, thyroid, thymic tissue, or lymph node) would result.[10–12]

This all changed with the development and implementation of the intraoperative parathyroid hormone (PTH) assay. The assay uses the knowledge of the kinetics of PTH, which has a half-life of 5 minutes. Hence, at the start of the surgery, a blood sample is obtained and sent to the laboratory for measurement of PTH; when the enlarged gland is identified and while frozen section analysis for confirmation of the abnormal parathyroid is taking place (usually with a 10- to 15-minute wait time from excision of the gland), a second blood sample is obtained and assayed. If the difference between the first and second assay results indicate an at least 50% drop in the level of hormone, the patient is considered cured. (Some experienced surgeons require that the second result be within the normal range for the assay used; this may reflect a drop of 75% or more from the initial hormone level [D.L. Fraker, personal communication, 2007].)[13–15]

EMBRYOLOGY AND LOCATION

The development of the parathyroid glands begins during the fifth to sixth weeks of embryologic life.[16–18] They travel and descend with the third and fourth pharyngeal pouches. Even here, the situation is not simple. Although it might be expected that the third pharyngeal pouch parathyroid is associated with superior glands and the fourth pouch with the lower, the opposite is true. Thus, the lower or inferior glands descend farther than the upper ones and are often associated with the thymus. Hence, parathyroid tissue may be present anywhere along the line of descent from the jaw to the pericardium.[16,19–22]

GROSS AND MICROANATOMY OF THE NORMAL PARATHYROID

The normal parathyroid gland is a kidney bean–shaped (reniform) structure whose weight ranges from 10 up to 55 mg, rarely heavier. The total weight of all the parathyroids is approximately 120 mg in men and 145 mg in women (however, up to a total weight of 200 mg has been considered within normal range).[16,17] The weight of the normal glands is dependent on gender, age, weight, and nutritional status of an individual.[23,24] The size of a normal gland is 4 to 6 mm long and 2 to 4 mm wide. It is red-brown in color and has a smooth outer surface. In some glands, the concentration of fat cells is such that small irregular nodules of yellow tissue admixed with the red brown parenchyma can be seen.

Parathyroid histology varies with age. Thus, in children, the parenchymal cells predominate and a ratio of cells to fat can be as high as 90%. In older individuals, that ratio may be as small as 10%, with a 50:50 ratio common in middle age (**Fig. 1**).[23,25] Pathologists must recognize, however, that the distribution of the parenchymal cells to fat cells is variable and, depending on the site of the gland sampled, the microscopic appearance may look atrophic (more than 90% fat cells) or hypercellular (more than 90% parenchymal cells). This variability has led to confusion with the microscopy of lesions in patients with clinical hyperfunction. This (discussed later) has been reflected in the literature, indicating that multigland "hyperplasia" accounts for more than 50% of primary hyperparathyroidism and that uniglandular adenomas are unusual.[3,26,27]

ATYPICAL LOCATIONS

Whether some locations of the parathyroids need to be considered atypical or merely a form of normal developmental variation can be debated. For surgeons and radiologists, however, and to a lesser extent pathologists, an understanding of where parathyroid tissue may be located is crucial

Fig. 1. (*A*) Normal para-thyroid gland in middle-aged (54-year-old) woman. Note ratio of parenchymal to flat cells is approximately 50:50 (H&E, original magnification ×20). (*B*) Higher magnification of A (H&E, original magnification ×100).

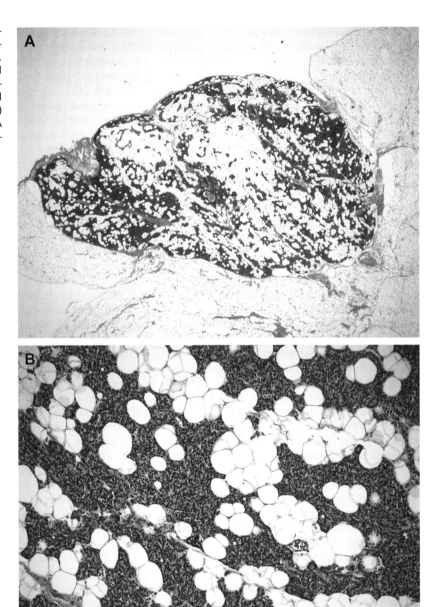

to locate hyperfunctioning gland(s) and lead to cure of the hyperparathyroidism.

From embryologic studies, a normal situation shows 1 parathyroid gland present at or close to each of the 4 poles of the thyroid gland. Because of under- or over-migration of the parathyroid tissue, however, some normal individuals have glands whose location is not normal. Hence, parathyroid tissue can be found within the thymus (either mediastinal or cervical), within the thyroid (although what appears to the surgeon as intra-thyroidal parathyroid may be a gland present within a nook or invagination of thyroid tissue and still microscopically be located outside of the thyroid), within the larynx, in the wall of the esophagus, behind the esophagus, in the carotid sheath, and in many other sites in the neck and upper mediastinum.[28–32]

It is critical to be aware that not all normal individuals have 4 parathyroid glands, although older careful autopsy studies indicate that approximately 85% of subjects do. In approximately 5% of cases, more than 4 glands are identified (usually 5, rarely more) and an equal number have only 3 glands. In some individuals, parathyroid tissue may not be organized into glands but as microscopic collections of parathyroid cells scattered within cervical fat or mediastinum.[21,33,34] This entity, known as parathyromatosis, is rarely, if ever, a clinical issue, except in patients with hyperfunctioning parathyroid tissue (ie, multigland hyperplasia), in which these microscopic cell nests are also involved in the process; hyperfunctional parathyroid tissue is thus present throughout the neck (parathyromatosis discussed later).

Functional histology of the glands is an important diagnostic factor. In euparathyroid individuals, approximately 80% of the parenchymal cells contain intracellular fat; in hyperfunction, this is lost or markedly decreased.[9,24,25,35–37] This has been beautifully documented by ultrastructural studies.[38] Thus, in the intraoperative situation, the use of fat stains can be helpful in recognition of the function of an individual parathyroid gland (or biopsy thereof) (Fig. 2). This fact can be used at the time of frozen section to guide surgeons and pathologists to normal versus abnormal parathyroid tissue.[5,36]

Each gland is enveloped by a delicate fibrous capsule, which extends into the gland dividing it into lobules. Each gland is supplied by a branch of the thyroid artery (either superior or inferior). Venous drainage is through branches of the thyroid arteries, and lymphatics empty through cervical channels into neck lymph nodes. The cytology of the parathyroid is basically the chief cells and its various disguises (clear cell and oncocyte) and the adipocyte. Oncocytes or oxyphil cells are virtually never found in parathyroids in children but begin to appear as individual cells or even micronodules after puberty.[39] Also, as are most endocrine tissues, the parathyroid gland is extremely vascular with a network of capillaries coursing through the entire structure.

PATHOLOGY

The surgical pathology of the parathyroid is essentially the pathology of hyperparathyroidism. Several entities are known to be responsible for hyperparathyroidism (Table 1); these are discussed later. The entities vary with the clinical type of hyperfunction: primary, secondary, and tertiary.

ADENOMA

Causes of parathyroid adenoma are not known but increasing numbers of reports indicate radiation to

the neck as a possible initiating event (Box 1). Thus, the coexistence of thyroid papillary carcinoma and parathyroid adenoma is higher than expected by chance; in addition, increasing numbers of cases of adenoma are reported in the population exposed to radiation at the time of the Chernobyl nuclear accident.[40–44]

It has become evident with increasing experience (including the use of intraoperative PTH assays) that primary hyperparathyroidism is caused by a single-gland adenoma in more than 80% of patients.[39,45,46] Clinically these individuals are often asymptomatic and discovered by routine biochemical screening or may have a history of mild symptoms, such as renal stones. There is a predominant female-to-male ratio of 3:1. Any gland may be affected although the lower ones are more commonly the site of adenoma.[39,46,47]

The approach to these patients is imaging (often ultrasound, radionuclide scan, or both) to identify the location of the offending gland. A surgical approach that is often minimally invasive is the next step and when the enlarged hyperfunctioning gland is removed, surgical cure is usually achieved. Long-term follow-up studies show that more than 95% of patients are rendered euparathyroid and cured with this surgery.[11,48]

These statistics belie the fact advanced approximately 3 decades ago[49] that approximately half of primary hyperparathyroidism is caused by multigland disease and that to cure the clinical condition, a 3.5-gland parathyroidectomy was required. This theory was related to pathologic misinterpretation of normal parathyroid morphologic variations wherein areas of some glands show concentrations of parenchymal cells and minimal extracellular adipose tissue leading to diagnoses of microscopic hyperplasia.

Parathyroid adenomas present as enlarged glands usually still maintaining the reniform shape of the normal parathyroid. The adenoma may weigh anywhere a few hundred milligrams to multiple grams.

Some studies have identified a correlation between the weight and size of the adenoma and the severity of hyperfunction.[39,45] It has been the authors' experience that many purely oncocytic adenomas (Fig. 3), however, may be of significant size (more than 1.5 g) and still show minimal elevation of serum calcium.[50]

The adenoma may have a capsule, which is usually very thin, and this separates it from the normal surrounding rim of normocellular parathyroid. Approximately 50% to 60% of adenomas demonstrate a rim.[39] The rim may not always be identified, however, either because of the method of sectioning of the adenoma or because the

Fig. 2. (*A*) Oil red O stain showing abundant red-staining intracellular far normal parathyroid gland (oil red O, original magnification ×40). (*B*) Same stain in adenoma (original magnification ×40).

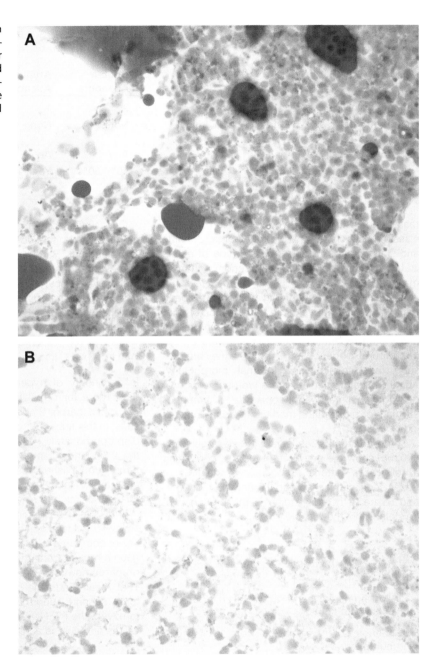

adenoma was so large as to obliterate the preexisting normal tissue. The tumor is often brown (usually darker than the normal gland) and soft. Microcysts may be present and rarely the adenoma may be predominantly cystic (discussed later).

Histologically, the adenoma shows a diffuse growth of the neoplastic cell and may show monotonous cellularity (usually chief cell) or a mixed cell type. The normal lobulation of the gland is no longer present. Prominent vascularity is seen

and on occasion small microhemorrhages may be noted.

Rarely, foci of spindle cell growth may be seen, although in the authors' experience this is more common in carcinomas. The nuclei of the tumor may be bland and monotonous or there may be areas of marked nuclear enlargement, hyperchromasia, and multinucleation. Such atypia (similar to so-called endocrine atypia seen in other endocrine organs) may be alarming (**Fig. 4**) but should be

Table 1
Pathologic key features parathyroid lesions associated with hyperparathyroidism

	Adenoma	Hyperplasia	Double Adenoma	Atypical Adenoma	Carcinoma
Glands involved	1	All	2	1	1
Associated lesions	None	Familial endocrine	None	None	HYPT–jaw tumor
Predominate cell	Any	Any	Any	Any	Any
Presence of rim	50%–60%	No	50%–60%	Yes	Often not
Invasion	No	No	No	Yes	Yes

reassuring in that it is a benign lesion. In their classic article on parathyroid carcinoma, Schantz and Castleman[51] warned that this type of atypia is found more commonly in adenoma than in malignancies.

Mitotic activity in parathyroid adenoma has been the subject of controversy. In the absence of prior trauma (such as an inadvertent aspiration biopsy) and thus a reparative phenomenon, mitoses are rarely found in adenomas. Certainly if they are present, they should show normal morphology. Abnormal mitotic figures are a worrisome sign of dealing with a malignant neoplasm.[51–54] Immunostaining for proliferation markers has shown a low index (<2%).[54–56]

Some adenomas, especially those larger than 800 mg, show the presence of follicles containing a colloid-like material. Especially at the time of frozen section; this may lead to confusion with thyroid tissue. A helpful finding is the presence of crystals within the "colloid."[1]

Box 1
Pathologic key points parathyroid pathology in hyperparathyroidism

1. Most primary hyperparathyroidism is due to solitary adenoma.

2. Adenomas can vary in size from 100 mg to multiple grams.

3. Double adenomas occur and are causes of between 3% and 7% of primary hyperparathyroidism.

4. Multigland disease may be synchronous or metasynchronous.

5. Metasynchronous cases of multigland disease can be mistaken for uniglandular adenoma.

6. Other lesions leading to primary hyperthyroidism, such as atypical adenoma, carcinoma, or cystic lesions, are rare and comprise approximately 5%–7%.

Occasional adenomas contain small nests of adipose tissue; this does not rule out a diagnosis of adenoma. Rarely, parathyroid proliferations and even normal glands have small collections of mature lymphocytes (**Fig. 5**). Some patients with this finding in their parathyroids also have chronic lymphocytic thyroiditis, suggesting an underlining immunologic association.[57–60]

DOUBLE ADENOMA

In a minority of hyperparathyroid patients who have more than 1 gland disease, approximately 3% to 5% harbor 2 adenomas.[61] For unclear reasons, in this subset of patients, the adenomas are disproportionately (48% in the authors' series) in the 2 superior glands, form the fourth branchial pouch (unpublished observations, 2010). Each adenoma taken alone has all the gross and histologic characteristics of a single adenoma.[62]

With the increasing use of intraoperative PTH assay, the identification of double adenoma is easier compared with historical experience. A surgeon removes 1 enlarged gland and the PTH level drops somewhat but not into the normal range. That result leads the surgeon to further explore for a second abnormal gland; once found and removed, the PTH level drops well into the normal values and cure is achieved.[12,63,64]

ATYPICAL ADENOMA

Rarely, 1 gland disease shows unusual morphologic features and is considered an atypical adenoma. The exact incidence of such lesions responsible for clinical hyperparathyroidism is unknown and, unfortunately, definitions vary. According to the World Health Organization (WHO, 2004)[65] definition, such glands are large and show either excess mitotic figures (not abnormal ones), invasion of the tumor capsule, and often the proliferation is divided by broad fibrous bands. There is no spontaneous tumor necrosis or vascular invasion, no invasion of nearby organs,

Fig. 3. Oncocytic para-thyroid adenoma. This gland weighed 2 g but serum calcium was only 10.0 mg/dL (H&E, original magnification ×10).

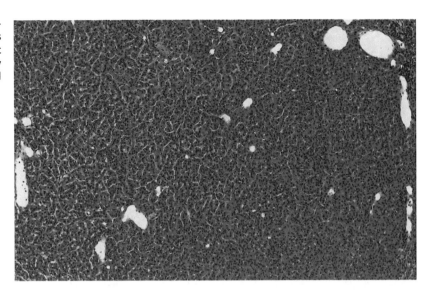

and no evidence of metastasis. Hence, the criteria for carcinoma are not met, but the features noted are beyond what is expected of a simple ade-noma. Although long-term follow-up data are still sparse on large numbers of such tumors, the infor-mation available suggests that most behave clini-cally in a benign fashion.[39,66,67]

CARCINOMA

Parathyroid carcinoma is a rare cause of hyper-parathyroidism, comprising approximately 1% or less of parathyroid neoplasms. Classically,[3,51,68–74] these lesions occur in patients somewhat younger than those with adenomas (indicating that ade-nomas probably do not transform into carcinomas), are associated with extremely elevation of serum calcium, and are often symptomatic.

Pathologically, carcinomas of the parathyroid are classically large tumors (may be multiple grams in weight), often adherent or invasive into neighboring structures or organs; experienced surgeons are suspicious of malignancy because of the operative findings. Histologically, the tumor grows in a sheetlike diffuse pattern of monotonous cells or may show significant pleomorphism; in some examples, spindle cell proliferation is found in parts of the tumor. Mitoses, including abnormal forms, are commonly seen and vascular invasion in the lesional capsule or in the surrounding soft tissue is also noted. Coagulative tumor necrosis is identified frequently.[3]

The diagnosis of malignancy, therefore, should be restricted to those cases that have evidence of invasion of adjacent soft tissues and associated structures, vascular channels, or perineural

spaces and/or to tumors with documented metas-tases. This view is also supported by the WHO.[65]

The cell makeup of carcinoma is usually the chief cell but oxyphilic tumors have also been described.[75] Occasionally, nonfunctioning parathy-roid carcinomas occur and these are often very large and obviously invasive tumors that have onco-cytic cytology. The differential diagnosis in these cases is with an oncocytic thyroid carcinoma (of either follicular or parafollicular C-cell origin), para-ganglioma or metastatic tumor (either neuroendo-cine type), or even malignant melanoma.

Parathyroid carcinomas that are functional are often indolent malignancies and have a long (20-year or longer) natural history. Metasta-ses to lung and bones are common, although regional lymph nodes, liver, and other organs can also be involved. Often, the cause of death may not be related to massive organ replace-ment but to the uncontrollable metabolic effects of the hypercalcemia.[68,70,72,75,76]

Nonfunctional carcinomas are particularly aggressive tumors compared with functioning neoplasms; the survival rate is short.[74–77] Although the cause of parathyroid carcinoma is unknown, there is one syndrome in which this tu-mor is frequently found—the hyperparathyroid-ism jaw tumor syndrome.[78–80] Approximately 15% of patients with this disorder develop para-thyroid carcinoma. The gene that normally en-codes for a protein parafibromin is mutated in this disease, leading to loss of expression of par-afibromin in the carcinomas. Immunostains for the protein can be performed and show loss of nuclear localization in the cancer. Extrapolating from this finding, Gill and colleagues[81] studied

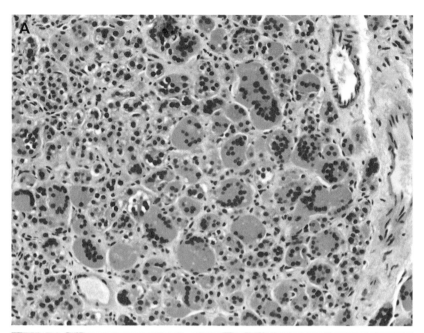

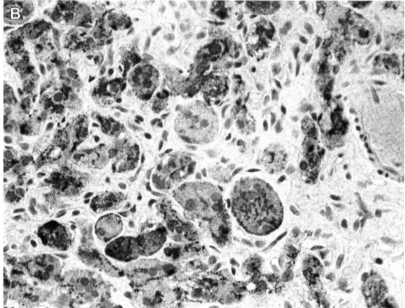

Fig. 4. (*A*) Parathyroid adenoma with monster giant cells. There were found multifocally in the lesion (H&E, original magnification ×10). (*B*) Immunostain for PTH proves these are parathyroid cells (PTH, original magnification ×20).

parafibromin immunolocalization in sporadic parathyroid adenomas and carcinomas. This group found that more than 90% of the 12 carcinomas they studied lost staining and 98% of adenomas retained nuclear positivity. Since the publication of that study, others have shown that parafibromin is lost in approximately 70% of sporadic parathyroid carcinomas and that it may also be lost in cystic adenomas and in parathyroid glands of patients with MEN type 1 (MEN1).[79,80,82–85]

Hyperplasia, Primary

Approximately 10% to 15% of primary hyperparathyroidism is caused by multigland (usually 4)

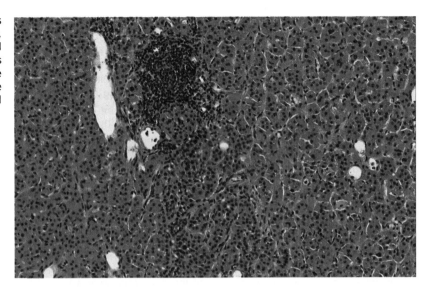

Fig. 5. Lymphocyte clusters can be seen in adenomas, hyperplasia, and normal parathyroid. Some patients with this finding have evidence of autoimmune thyroiditis (H&E, original magnification ×20).

hyperplasia, wherein all the parathyroid tissue is abnormally cellular and functioning, the glands are enlarged (either symmetrically or asymmetrically), and fat stain indicates that all the tissue shows decreased or absent intracellular fat (**Box 2**). The glands may show a diffuse proliferation of parenchymal cells with little or no extracellular fat of they may be nodular; the individual nodules are usually of chief cell type although foci of oncocytes and clear cells may be admixed.[3]

This 4-gland disease may be seen sporadically. In some cases, 1 gland may be asymmetrically enlarged and the surgeon may assume this is a solitary adenoma (in the age of intraoperative hormone assay; however, this scenario is less common because the hormone level may not drop as expected in uniglandular disease). This lesion, however, is the commonly found in familial hyperparathyroidism and in MEN syndromes (especially MEN1 or Wermer syndrome).[3,86–89]

Pathologically, all 4 glands are enlarged although occasionally 1 may be marked bigger than the others. Microscopically, the glands are hypercellular and can show nodularity (rarely, some nodules show fibrous capsules and even dystrophic calcification). The cell type is predominantly chief cell although mixed cell nodules with oxyphils and clear cells can be found.[3,86] Mitoses can be seen.[3,90]

The surgical approach is one of total paratyroidectomy with reimplantation of a portion of 1 gland (often in the muscle of the arm) and preservation of some parathyroid tissue in the event of hypocalcemia (if the implant does not take). Some surgeons prefer 3.5-gland excision with marking the residual half gland remaining in the event that titration of the serum calcium is needed in the future.[91–93]

A truly rare entity is known as clear cell hyperplasia wherein all 4 glands are enlarged (often huge) and the upper glands are larger than the lower (this is different from other forms of hyperplasia).[94–97]

Secondary Hyperplasia

In contrast to primary hyperplasia wherein a stimulus to the parathyroid mass is unknown, in secondary hyperparathyroidism, a known stimulus is present; in North America, this is overwhelmingly chronic renal failure. The relationship between chronic renal failure and enlargement of multiple parathyroid glands has been known for many years. Overproduction of PTH and parathyroid proliferation in this setting result from hyperphosphatemia, low levels of ionized calcium in the blood, and impaired 1,25-dihydroxyvitamin D synthesis by the diseased kidneys. When plasma levels of calcium decrease, the calcium sensing

---

Box 2
Pathologic points primary hyperthyroidism

The causes of recurrent hyperthyroidism include

1. Mistaking multigland disease (including double adenoma) for 1 gland lesion (metasynchronous gland involvement)

2. Spillage of an abnormal gland during removal leading to parathyromatosis

3. Underdiagnoses of parathyroid carcinoma

4. Presence of primary parathyromatosis

receptor (CaSR) responds by increasing the secretion of PTH, resulting in a compensatory mechanism to restore normal function.[18,98,99]

Secondary hyperparathyroidism may also occur in patients with deficiency of vitamin D, abnormal vitamin D metabolism, or malabsorptive states or after the administration of certain drugs (eg, lithium). Once the process of parathyroid hyperplasia begins, the set point for the control of PTH secretion by ionized calcium rises and this leads to further hyperplasia of the glands and hypersecretion of PTH.[100–103]

The pathology is that all 4 glands are enlarged, usually nodular and with absent or decreased extra- and intracellular fat. The nodules may be composed of chief cells, oxyphils or oncocytes, and clear cells; often, mixed cellularity is present. Mitoses can be found but not abnormal forms. Pleomorphism is rare. In some cases, 1 of the 4 glands is markedly larger than the other 3, but more often the enlargement is uniform.[3,104]

Tertiary Hyperparathyroidism

The tertiary form of hyperfunction occurs in patients with chronic renal failure in whom on a background of secondary hyperplasia, 1 gland or a portion of 1 gland becomes autonomously functioning. In addition, this entity may manifest as recurrent hyperparathyroidism after successful treatment of secondary form and of the underlying renal disease.[105–107]

Unusual Lesions

Cysts

Microscopic cysts in normal or hyperfunctional parathyroid glands are not rare, but grossly cystic glands are. The cysts are thin walled and contain clear fluid, which is pure PTH. Such lesions may be associated with hyperparathyroidism and many authors consider that these represent cystic parathyroid adenomas.[108–110]

Cystic change in multiple hyperplastic glands can be found in the setting of MEN1 (Wermer syndrome) and in the hyperparathyroidism–jaw tumor syndrome (associated with mutations in the gene that encodes for parafibromin).[111,112]

Parathyromatosis

The term, *parathyromatosis*, refers to the presence of multiple nodules of hypercellular functioning parathyroid tissue beyond the confines of the normal parathyroid glands. In primary parathyromatosis, developmental rests of parathyroid tissue occur in the soft tissues of the neck and mediastinum, including within the thymus. In patients with primary or secondary hyperplasia wherein all the parathyroid tissue is affected,

these rests may also become hyperplastic; this is then responsible for persistent or recurrent hyperparathyroidism. In the setting of primary hyperplasia, it has been the authors' experience that this disorder is most commonly seen in the setting of MEN1.

A second mechanism for the development of parathyromatosis is seeding of the operative field during parathyroidectomy or incomplete excision of hyperplastic or neoplastic parathyroid lesions (secondary parathyromatosis); in the authors' experience, this is most often found in the setting of spillage of a large gland in patients with renal failure–associated hyperparathyroidism.[113–115]

The pathologic differential diagnosis of parathyromatosis is with parathyroid carcinoma. In the primary form, the multiplicity of the nodules and their smooth outline without associated fibrosis is a helpful histologic clue. In secondary parathyromatosis, the prior surgery may cause fibrosis, the spillage may be into skeletal muscle and fat, simulating invasion, and mitotic activity may be found. All these microscopic findings are identical to what is found in parathyroid transplants. Helpful diagnostic clues to distinguish this lesion from carcinoma include the absence of abnormal mitotic figures or vascular invasion and the smooth outline of the nodules.[34,116,117]

Lipoadenoma

A rare tumor of the parathyroid, the lipoadenoma, may be associated with hyperfunction. It is composed of fat and hypercellular parenchyma. Often large (up to several hundred grams), the function of these lesions may be due to the increased parenchymal mass of chief cells and not the fat. Some examples have contained myxoid stroma as well as fat.[118–121]

Metastases to parathyroid

Although the parathyroids are very vascular organs, metastatic disease to them is rare. Autopsy studies have disclosed anywhere from 2% to 11% of patients dying of disseminated cancer show metastases to 1 or more parathyroids. In the modern era with many cancer patients surviving for longer periods of time, surgical specimens of parathyroid glands containing metastases may be seen with increasing frequency. (The authors' group has seen 3 such cases in the past year.) The primary sites for the metastatic lesions include breast, lung, neuroendocrine carcinomas, and kidney. The last of these could be problematic because kidney carcinoma often shows clear cell cytology and both renal carcinoma and parathyroid tissue can show positive immunostaining for renal cell carcinoma (RCC) antigen.[122–127]

Post–Fine-Needle Aspiration Changes

Although the parathyroid is not a site that is often targeted for aspiration biopsy, on occasion in the workup of an assumed thyroid nodule, a parathyroid gland or lesion may be inadvertently sampled. In addition, intrathyroidal parathyroids may be targeted as thyroid nodules. Hence, cytopathologists must be aware of this possibility and, if parathyroid tissue is suspected (due to monotony of cell proliferation, vascularity, and small round regular nuclei), an additional sample or a rinse of the needle can be obtained and submitted for PTH assay.[128–131] If cell block material is available, immunostaining for PTH (if available), chromogranin A (positive), and thyroid transcription factor-1 (negative) can be diagnostically useful.

Unfortunately, as a consequence of the fine-needle aspiration trauma, the parathyroid lesion may undergo changes, such as infarction (which, if total, cures the metabolic abnormality) or fibrosis leading to a pseudoinvasive picture. The presence of linear geographic fibrosis and hemosiderin in the setting of an appropriate history usually resolves the issue.[6]

Immunostains

Parathyroid hormone
Parathyroid tissue, whether normal or abnormal, shows the presence of PTH in the cytoplasm. This stain is useful in those questionable situations wherein the histologic identification by H&E stain alone is doubtful. Oncocytes tend to stain less strongly than chief cells.[39,77,132]

Chromogranin A and synaptophysin
The markers, chromogranin A and synaptophysin, are in common use in many histology laboratories (in contrast to antibodies to PTH). Parathyroid cells contain both proteins and these stains can be helpful in those proliferations wherein a follicular pattern is prominent. Follicular thyroid tissue is nonreactive.[3,39,133] (The experience in the authors' laboratory favors using chromogranin staining and not using synaptophysin.)

Calcitonin and the calcitonin gene–related peptide
Calcitonin and the calcitonin gene–related peptide are synthesized and stored in a small subset of hyperplastic parathyroid cells.[134]

Renal cell carcinoma
RCC antigen first identified in kidney cancer has been shown to stain approximately 100% of parathyroid lesions as well as the normal glands. It can be helpful if the distinction between thyroid and parathyroid tissue is needed.[135,136]

Thyroid transcription factor-1
Thyroid transcription factor-1 is found in many tissues and tumors (thyroid, lung, reproductive organs, and so forth). It is, however, negative in parathyroid tissue and, again, in that rare situation where distinguishing thyroid from parathyroid is important, this marker can be helpful in a panel of stains, including chromogranin and PTH.

Parafibromin
The parafibromin protein, a product of the HRPT2/CDC73 gene, is expressed within the nuclei of normal chief cells.[79,81] It is retained in normal and most benign parathyroid lesions and is classically lost in carcinomas. Originally reported as 95% specific for malignancy,[81] subsequent studies have shown it is less helpful than that (approximately 70% of cases).[137–139]

PAX8
PAX8 immunoreactivity is present in approximately one-third of normal parathyroid glands.[140]

Proliferation markers
Ki67 can be used in those instances wherein by tumor size or weight, a parathyroid lesion is concerning for malignancy or atypia. A proliferation index of greater than 2% is worrisome and should be listed in the pathology report. Some early studies indicated that a higher than 5% index might be helpful in predicting recurrence in hyperplastic glands in 4-gland disease.[54,141–143]

A BIT ABOUT MOLECULAR BIOLOGY

Germline mutations of the HRPT2/CDC73 gene, which encodes parafibromin (a protein that inhibits cell proliferation and promotes apoptosis), are responsible for the development of parathyroid carcinoma in the hyperparathyroidism–jaw tumor syndrome.[79] Somatic mutations of this gene also occur in approximately 70% of sporadic parathyroid carcinomas. Sporadic adenomas rarely harbor HRPT2/CDC73 mutations[144]; they do not play a significant role in the development of these common neoplasms.[144–147]

Early studies reported that most parathyroid carcinomas lacked a retinoblastoma (RB) allele.[148] In one study, loss of heterozygosity for at least 1 marker of the RB allele was found in all parathyroid carcinomas and in 28% of adenomas.[149] Further analyses showed no significant molecular events in RB gene; hence, it is now believed that RB is unlikely to act as a tumor suppressor gene and have a role in the development of parathyroid carcinomas. The RB protein is present in most adenomas.[56]

CaSR mRNA is significantly reduced in adenomas compared with normal glands. These findings suggest that the lowered levels of CaSR mRNA in adenomas may contribute to the increased set point of PTH secretion. Reduction of CaSR has also been reported in adenomas from patients with secondary hyperparathyroidism.[150–153]

Loss of the adenomatous polyposis gene coli product (APC) immunoreactivity and reduced expression of parafibromin have been reported in 40% of atypical parathyroid adenomas whereas usual parathyroid adenomas are positive for these markers.[154,155]

MOLECULAR GENETIC FEATURES

Early studies, based on glucose-6-phosphate dehydrogenase isoenzyme patterns, indicated that parathyroid adenomas were polyclonal proliferations. Subsequent analyses, however, have revealed that a vast majority of parathyroid adenomas are clonal lesions, as demonstrated by X-chromosome inactivation and DNA polymorphism studies.[156,157] Both the parathyroid adenoma (PRAD1)/cyclin D1 (CCND1) and MEN1 genes have been implicated in the development of these tumors.[41,44,158–160]

Mutations of the MEN1 gene (11q13), which encodes menin, are responsible for the development of the MEN1 syndrome.[161,162] Loss of one MEN1 allele also occurs in up to 40% of sporadic parathyroid adenomas with an inactivating mutation in the other allele occurring in approximately 50% of these cases.[41,163–168] It has been suggested that the inactivation of the MEN1 gene is an important genetic alteration in radiation-induced parathyroid adenomas.[165]

SUMMARY

This review focuses on the pathology of parathyroid in hyperparathyroidism. Lesions associated with this metabolic disorder, including adenoma, atypical adenoma, carcinoma, and hyperplasia, are discussed. The associations of some parathyroid disorders with specific genetic syndromes are also reviewed. Unusual lesions of the parathyroids are briefly described. Ancillary techniques that may be useful in the distinction of these various parathyroid proliferations are also included.

REFERENCES

1. Westra WH, Pritchett DD, Udelsman R. Intraoperative confirmation of parathyroid tissue during parathyroid exploration: a retrospective evaluation of the frozen section. Am J Surg Pathol 1998;22: 538–44.

2. Baloch ZW, LiVolsi VA. Intraoperative assessment of thyroid and parathyroid lesions. Semin Diagn Pathol 2002;19:219–26.

3. Baloch ZW, LiVolsi VA. Pathology of the parathyroid glands in hyperparathyroidism. Semin Diagn Pathol 2013;30:165–77.

4. Morris LF, Zanocco K, Ituarte PH, et al. The value of intraoperative parathyroid hormone monitoring in localized primary hyperparathyroidism: a cost analysis. Ann Surg Oncol 2010;17:679–85.

5. Roth SI, Faquin WC. The pathologist's intraoperative role during parathyroid surgery. Arch Pathol Lab Med 2003;127:15.

6. Alwaheeb S, Rambaldini G, Boerner S, et al. Worrisome histologic alterations following fine-needle aspiration of the parathyroid. J Clin Pathol 2006; 59:1094–6.

7. Carpenter JM, Michaelson PG, Lidner TK, et al. Parathyromatosis. Ear Nose Throat J 2007;86:21.

8. Akerstrom G, Rudberg C, Grimelius L, et al. Histologic parathyroid abnormalities in an autopsy series. Hum Pathol 1986;17:520–7.

9. Roth SI, Gallagher MJ. The rapid identification of "normal" parathyroid glands by the presence of intracellular fat. Am J Pathol 1976;84:521–8.

10. Wang CA, Rieder SV. A density test for the intraoperative differentiation of parathyroid hyperplasia from neoplasia. Ann Surg 1978;187:63–7.

11. Miccoli P, Bendinelli C, Berti P, et al. Video-assisted versus conventional parathyroidectomy in primary hyperparathyroidism: a prospective randomized study. Surgery 1999;126:1117–21 [discussion: 1121–2].

12. Greene AB, Butler RS, McIntyre S, et al. National trends in parathyroid surgery from 1998 to 2008: a decade of change. J Am Coll Surg 2009;209:332–43.

13. Monchik JM, Barellini L, Langer P, et al. Minimally invasive parathyroid surgery in 103 patients with local/regional anesthesia, without exclusion criteria. Surgery 2002;131:502–8.

14. Udelsman R. Primary hyperparathyroidism. Curr Treat Options Oncol 2001;2:365–72.

15. Irvin GL 3rd, Deriso GT 3rd. A new, practical intraoperative parathyroid hormone assay. Am J Surg 1994;168:466–8.

16. Grimelius L, Akerstrom G, Johansson H, et al. Anatomy and histopathology of human parathyroid glands. Pathol Annu 1981;16:1–24.

17. Hunt PS, Poole M, Reeve TS. A reappraisal of the surgical anatomy of the thyroid and parathyroid glands. Br J Surg 1968;55:63–6.

18. Butterworth PC, Nicholson ML. Surgical anatomy of the parathyroid glands in secondary hyperparathyroidism. J R Coll Surg Edinb 1998;43:271–3.

19. Thompson NW, Eckhauser FE, Harness JK. The anatomy of primary hyperparathyroidism. Surgery 1982;92:814–21.

20. Lengele B, Hamoir M. Anatomy and embryology of the parathyroid glands. Acta Otorhinolaryngol Belg 2001;55:89–93.

21. Reddick RL, Costa JC, Marx SJ. Parathyroid hyperplasia and parathyromatosis. Lancet 1977;1:549.

22. Akerstrom G, Malmaeus J, Grimelius L, et al. Histological changes in parathyroid glands in subclinical and clinical renal disease. An autopsy investigation. Scand J Urol Nephrol 1984;18:75–84.

23. Dufour DR, Wilkerson SY. The normal parathyroid revisited: percentage of stromal fat. Hum Pathol 1982;13:717–21.

24. Dekker A, Dunsford HA, Geyer SJ. The normal parathyroid gland at autopsy: the significance of stromal fat in adult patients. J Pathol 1979;128:127–32.

25. Dufour DR, Durkowski C. Sudan IV stain. Its limitations in evaluating parathyroid functional status. Arch Pathol Lab Med 1982;106:224–7.

26. Kebebew E, Hwang J, Reiff E, et al. Predictors of single-gland vs multigland parathyroid disease in primary hyperparathyroidism: a simple and accurate scoring model. Arch Surg 2006;141:777–82 [discussion: 782].

27. Awad SS, Miskulin J, Thompson N. Parathyroid adenomas versus four-gland hyperplasia as the cause of primary hyperparathyroidism in patients with prolonged lithium therapy. World J Surg 2003;27:486–8.

28. Yeh MW, Barraclough BM, Sidhu SB, et al. Two hundred consecutive parathyroid ultrasound studies by a single clinician: the impact of experience. Endocr Pract 2006;12:257–63.

29. Graff-Baker A, Roman SA, Boffa D, et al. Diagnosis of ectopic middle mediastinal parathyroid adenoma using endoscopic ultrasonography-guided fine-needle aspiration with real-time rapid parathyroid hormone assay. J Am Coll Surg 2009;209:e1–4.

30. Ogus M, Mayir B, Dinckan A. Mediastinal, cystic and functional parathyroid adenoma in patients with double parathyroid adenomas: a case report. Acta Chir Belg 2006;106:736–8.

31. Pitsilos SA, Weber R, Baloch Z, et al. Ectopic parathyroid adenoma initially suspected to be a thyroid lesion. Arch Pathol Lab Med 2002;126:1541–2.

32. Salem C, Massiani MA, Bazot M, et al. Retrotracheal cystic mass in the mediastinum. Rev Pneumol Clin 2002;58:226–31 [in French].

33. Tublin ME, Yim JH, Carty SE. Recurrent hyperparathyroidism secondary to parathyromatosis: clinical and imaging findings. J Ultrasound Med 2007;26:847–51.

34. Baloch ZW, Fraker D, LiVolsi VA. Parathyromatosis as cause of recurrent secondary hyperparathyroidism: a cytologic diagnosis. Diagn Cytopathol 2001;25:403–5.

35. Ljungberg T, Ungerstedt U. Evidence that the different properties of haloperidol and clozapine are not explained by differences in anticholinergic potency. Psychopharmacology 1979;60:303–7.

36. Bondeson AG, Bondeson L, Ljungberg O, et al. Fat staining in parathyroid disease–diagnostic value and impact on surgical strategy: clinicopathologic analysis of 191 cases. Hum Pathol 1985;16:1255–63.

37. Kasdon EJ, Rosen S, Cohen RB, et al. Surgical pathology of hyperparathyroidism. Usefulness of fat stain and problems in interpretation. Am J Surg Pathol 1981;5:381–4.

38. Cinti S, Sbarbati A. Ultrastructure of human parathyroid cells in health and disease. Microsc Res Tech 1995;32:164–79.

39. DeLellis RA, editor. Tumors of parathyroid gland. Washington, DC: Armed Forces Institute of Pathology; 1993.

40. Livolsi VA, Feind CR. Incidental medullary thyroid carcinoma in sporadic hyperparathyroidism. An expansion of the concept of C-cell hyperplasia. Am J Clin Pathol 1979;71:595–9.

41. Arnold A, Shattuck TM, Mallya SM, et al. Molecular pathogenesis of primary hyperparathyroidism. J Bone Miner Res 2002;17(Suppl 2):N30–6.

42. Bakker B, van der Eerden BC, Koppenaal DW, et al. Effect of x-irradiation on growth and the expression of parathyroid hormone-related peptide and Indian hedgehog in the tibial growth plate of the rat. Horm Res 2003;59:35–41.

43. Boehm BO, Rosinger S, Belyi D, et al. The parathyroid as a target for radiation damage. N Engl J Med 2011;365:676–8.

44. Hendy GN. Molecular mechanisms of primary hyperparathyroidism. Rev Endocr Metab Disord 2000;1:297–305.

45. Castleman B, Roth SI, editors. Tumors of the parathyroid glands. Washington, DC: Armed Forces Institute of Pathology; 1978.

46. Marcocci C, Cetani F. Clinical practice. Primary hyperparathyroidism. N Engl J Med 2011;365:2389–97.

47. Woolner LB, Keating FR Jr, Black BM. Tumors and hyperplasia of the parathyroid glands; a review of the pathological findings in 140 cases of primary hyperparathyroidism. Cancer 1952;5:1069–88.

48. Gooding GA, Duh QY. Primary hyperparathyroidism: functioning hemorrhagic parathyroid cyst. J Clin Ultrasound 1997;25:82–4.

49. Prinz RA, Lonchyna V, Carnaille B, et al. Thoracoscopic excision of enlarged mediastinal parathyroid glands. Surgery 1994;116:999–1004 [discussion: 1004–5].

50. Bedetti CD, Dekker A, Watson CG. Functioning oxyphil cell adenoma of the parathyroid gland: a clinicopathologic study of ten patients with hyperparathyroidism. Hum Pathol 1984;15:1121–6.

51. Schantz A, Castleman B. Parathyroid carcinoma. A study of 70 cases. Cancer 1973;31:600–5.

52. Snover DC, Foucar K. Mitotic activity in benign para-thyroid disease. Am J Clin Pathol 1981;75:345–7.

53. Sanjuan X, Bryant BR, Sobel ME, et al. Clonality analysis of benign parathyroid lesions by human androgen receptor (HUMARA) gene assay. Endocr Pathol 1998;9:293–300.

54. Tokumoto M, Tsuruya K, Fukuda K, et al. Reduced p21, p27 and vitamin D receptor in the nodular hyperplasia in patients with advanced secondary hyperparathyroidism. Kidney Int 2002;62:1196–207.

55. Alo PL, Visca P, Mazzaferro S, et al. Immunohistochemical study of fatty acid synthase, Ki67, proliferating cell nuclear antigen, and p53 expression in hyperplastic parathyroids. Ann Diagn Pathol 1999;3:287–93.

56. Lloyd RV, Carney JA, Ferreiro JA, et al. Immunohistochemical analysis of the cell cycle-associated antigens Ki-67 and retinoblastoma protein in parathyroid carcinomas and adenomas. Endocr Pathol 1995;6:279–87.

57. Varma D, Nigam S, Singhal N, et al. A report of two cases of Hashimoto's thyroiditis and synchronous parathyroid adenoma. Indian J Pathol Microbiol 2006;49:635–6.

58. Ebrahimi H, Edhouse P, Lundgren CI, et al. Does autoimmune thyroid disease affect parathyroid autotransplantation and survival? ANZ J Surg 2009; 79:383–5.

59. Auger M, Charbonneau M, Huttner I. Unsuspected intrathyroidal parathyroid adenoma: mimic of lymphocytic thyroiditis in fine-needle aspiration specimens-a case report. Diagn Cytopathol 1999; 21:276–9.

60. Gittes RF. Experimental autoimmune thyroiditis in transplanted isologous tissue and attempts to produce parathyroid lesions. Clin Exp Immunol 1966; 1:297–306.

61. Tezelman S, Shen W, Shaver JK, et al. Double parathyroid adenomas. Clinical and biochemical characteristics before and after parathyroidectomy. Ann Surg 1993;218:300–7 [discussion: 307–9].

62. Harness JK, Ramsburg SR, Nishiyama RH, et al. Multiple adenomas of the parathyroids: do they exist? Arch Surg 1979;114:468–74.

63. Mitchell J, Milas M, Barbosa G, et al. Avoidable reoperations for thyroid and parathyroid surgery: effect of hospital volume. Surgery 2008;144: 899–906 [discussion: 906–7].

64. Sharma J, Milas M, Berber E, et al. Value of intraoperative parathyroid hormone monitoring. Ann Surg Oncol 2008;15:493–8.

65. DeLellis RA, Lloyd RD, Heitz PU, et al. WHO: pathology and genetics. In: Kleihues P, Sobin LE, editors. Tumours of endocrine organs. Lyon (France): IARC Press; 2004. p. 493–8.

66. Stojadinovic A, Hoos A, Nissan A, et al. Parathyroid neoplasms: clinical, histopathological, and tissue microarray-based molecular analysis. Hum Pathol 2003;34:54–64.

67. Fernandez-Ranvier GG, Khanafshar E, Jensen K, et al. Parathyroid carcinoma, atypical parathyroid adenoma, or parathyromatosis? Cancer 2007;110: 255–64.

68. Agrawal R, Agarwal A, Kar DK, et al. Parathyroid carcinoma. J Assoc Physicians India 2001;49:990–3.

69. Bell WC. Surgical pathology of the parathyroid glands. Adv Exp Med Biol 2005;563:1–9.

70. Beus KS, Stack BC Jr. Parathyroid carcinoma. Otolaryngol Clin North Am 2004;37:845–54.

71. Bornstein-Quevedo L, Gamboa-Dominguez A, Angeles-Angeles A, et al. Histologic diagnosis of primary hyperparathyroidism: a concordance analysis between three pathologists. Endocr Pathol 2001;12:49–54.

72. Busaidy NL, Jimenez C, Habra MA, et al. Parathyroid carcinoma: a 22-year experience. Head Neck 2004;26:716–26.

73. Owen RP, Silver CE, Pellitteri PK, et al. Parathyroid carcinoma: a review. Head Neck 2011;33:429–36.

74. Fang SH, Lal G. Parathyroid cancer. Endocr Pract 2011;17(Suppl 1):36–43.

75. Erickson LA, Jin L, Papotti M, et al. Oxyphil parathyroid carcinomas: a clinicopathologic and immunohistochemical study of 10 cases. Am J Surg Pathol 2002;26:344–9.

76. Abdelgadir Adam M, Untch BR, Olson JA Jr. Parathyroid carcinoma: current understanding and new insights into gene expression and intraoperative parathyroid hormone kinetics. Oncologist 2010; 15:61–72.

77. Botea V, Edelson GW, Munasinghe RL. Hyperparathyroidism, hypercalcemia, and calcified brain metastatic lesions in a patient with small cell carcinoma demonstrating positive immunostain for parathyroid hormone. Endocr Pract 2003;9:40–4.

78. Carlson D. Parathyroid pathology: hyperparathyroidism and parathyroid tumors. Arch Pathol Lab Med 2010;134:1639–44.

79. Carpten JD, Robbins CM, Villablanca A, et al. HRPT2, encoding parafibromin, is mutated in hyperparathyroidism-jaw tumor syndrome. Nat Genet 2002;32:676–80.

80. Bradley KJ, Cavaco BM, Bowl MR, et al. Parafibromin mutations in hereditary hyperparathyroidism syndromes and parathyroid tumours. Clin Endocrinol 2006;64:299–306.

81. Gill AJ, Clarkson A, Gimm O, et al. Loss of nuclear expression of parafibromin distinguishes parathyroid carcinomas and hyperparathyroidism-jaw tumor (HPT-JT) syndrome-related adenomas from sporadic parathyroid adenomas and hyperplasias. Am J Surg Pathol 2006;30:1140–9.

82. Tan MH, Morrison C, Wang P, et al. Loss of parafibromin immunoreactivity is a distinguishing feature

of parathyroid carcinoma. Clin Cancer Res 2004; 10:6629–37.

83. Rozenblatt-Rosen O, Hughes CM, Nannepaga SJ, et al. The parafibromin tumor suppressor protein is part of a human Paf1 complex. Mol Cell Biol 2005;25:612–20.

84. Farber LJ, Kort EJ, Wang P, et al. The tumor suppressor parafibromin is required for posttranscriptional processing of histone mRNA. Mol Carcinog 2010;49:215–23.

85. Wang O, Wang C, Nie M, et al. Novel HRPT2/CDC73 gene mutations and loss of expression of parafibromin in Chinese patients with clinically sporadic parathyroid carcinomas. PLoS One 2012;7: e45567.

86. DeLellis RA, Mazzaglia P, Mangray S. Primary hyperparathyroidism: a current perspective. Arch Pathol Lab Med 2008;132:1251–62.

87. DeLellis RA. The neuroendocrine system and its tumors: an overview. Am J Clin Pathol 2001; 115(Suppl):S5–16.

88. Karges W, Jostarndt K, Maier S, et al. Multiple endocrine neoplasia type 1 (MEN1) gene mutations in a subset of patients with sporadic and familial primary hyperparathyroidism target the coding sequence but spare the promoter region. J Endocrinol 2000;166:1–9.

89. Dwarakanathan AA, Zwart S, Oathus RC. Isolated familial hyperparathyroidism with a novel mutation of the MEN1 gene. Endocr Pract 2000;6:268–70.

90. Chaitin BA, Goldman RL. Mitotic activity in benign parathyroid disease. Am J Clin Pathol 1981;76:363–4.

91. Agarwal G, Barraclough BH, Reeve TS, et al. Minimally invasive parathyroidectomy using the 'focused' lateral approach. II. Surgical technique. ANZ J Surg 2002;72:147–51.

92. Alveryd A. Parathyroid glands in thyroid surgery. I. Anatomy of parathyroid glands. II. Postoperative hypoparathyroidism–identification and autotransplantation of parathyroid glands. Acta Chir Scand 1968;389:1–120.

93. Calo PG, Pisano G, Loi G, et al. Surgery for primary hyperparathyroidism in patients with preoperatively negative sestamibi scan and discordant imaging studies: the usefulness of intraoperative parathyroid hormone monitoring. Clin Med Insights Endocrinol Diabetes 2013;6:63–7.

94. Tominaga Y, Grimelius L, Johansson H, et al. Histological and clinical features of non-familial primary parathyroid hyperplasia. Pathol Res Pract 1992; 188:115–22.

95. Absher KJ, Truong LD, Khurana KK, et al. Parathyroid cytology: avoiding diagnostic pitfalls. Head Neck 2002;24:157–64.

96. Sheldon H. On the water-clear cell in the human parathyroid gland. J Ultrastruct Res 1964;10: 377–83.

97. Stout LC Jr. Water-clear-cell hyperplasia mimicking parathyroid adenoma. Hum Pathol 1985;16:1075–6.

98. Malmaeus J, Grimelius L, Johansson H, et al. Parathyroid pathology in hyperparathyroidism secondary to chronic renal failure. Scand J Urol Nephrol 1984;18:157–66.

99. Jimeno J, Perez M, Pereira JA, et al. Surgical treatment of recurrent secondary hyperparathyroidism. Cir Esp 2005;78:34–8 [in Spanish].

100. Silver J, Kilav R, Naveh-Many T. Mechanisms of secondary hyperparathyroidism. Am J Phys 2002; 283:F367–76.

101. Goodman WG. Calcimimetic agents and secondary hyperparathyroidism: treatment and prevention. Nephrol Dial Transplant 2002;17:204–7.

102. Falvo L, Catania A, Sorrenti S, et al. Relapsing secondary hyperparathyroidism due to multiple nodular formations after total parathyroidectomy with autograft. Am Surg 2003;69:998–1002.

103. Eid W, Wheeler TM, Sharma MD. Recurrent hypercalcemia due to ectopic production of parathyroid hormone-related protein and intact parathyroid hormone in a single patient with multiple malignancies. Endocr Pract 2004;10:125–8.

104. Yamasaki K. Pathology of renal secondary hyperparathyroidism in mice. Jikken Dobutsu 1986;35:93–6.

105. Dorenbeck U, Leingartner T, Bretschneider T, et al. Tentorial and dural calcification with tertiary hyperparathyroidism: a rare entity in chronic renal failure. Eur Radiol 2002;12(Suppl 3):S11–3.

106. Rivkees SA, el-Hajj-Fuleihan G, Brown EM, et al. Tertiary hyperparathyroidism during high phosphate therapy of familial hypophosphatemic rickets. J Clin Endocrinol Metab 1992;75:1514–8.

107. Sharma J, Bajpai A, Kabra M, et al. Hypocalcemia clinical, biochemical, radiological profile and follow-up in a tertiary hospital in India. Indian Pediatr 2002;39:276–82.

108. Jarnagin WR, Clark OH. Mediastinal parathyroid cyst causing persistent hyperparathyroidism: case report and review of the literature. Surgery 1998;123:709–11.

109. Fortson JK, Patel VG, Henderson VJ. Parathyroid cysts: a case report and review of the literature. Laryngoscope 2001;111:1726–8.

110. Ippolito G, Palazzo FF, Sebag F, et al. A single-institution 25-year review of true parathyroid cysts. Langenbecks Arch Surg 2006;391:13–8.

111. Mallette LE, Malini S, Rappaport MP, et al. Familial cystic parathyroid adenomatosis. Ann Intern Med 1987;107:54–60.

112. Villablanca A, Farnebo F, Teh BT, et al. Genetic and clinical characterization of sporadic cystic parathyroid tumours. Clin Endocrinol 2002;56:261–9.

113. Palmer JA, Brown WA, Kerr WH, et al. The surgical aspects of hyperparathyroidism. Arch Surg 1975; 110:1004–7.

114. Fitko R, Roth SI, Hines JR, et al. Parathyromatosis in hyperparathyroidism. Hum Pathol 1990;21:234–7.

115. Lee PC, Mateo RB, Clarke MR, et al. Parathyromatosis: a cause for recurrent hyperparathyroidism. Endocr Pract 2001;7:189–92.

116. Lentsch EJ, Withrow KP, Ackermann D, et al. Parathyromatosis and recurrent hyperparathyroidism. Arch Otolaryngol Head Neck Surg 2003;129:894–6.

117. Bisceglia M, Spagnolo D, Galliani C, et al. Tumoral, quasitumoral and pseudotumoral lesions of the superficial and somatic soft tissue: new entities and new variants of old entities recorded during the last 25 years. Part XII: appendix. Pathologica 2006;98:239–98.

118. Weiland LH, Garrison RC, ReMine WH, et al. Lipoadenoma of the parathyroid gland. Am J Surg Pathol 1978;2:3–7.

119. Turner WJ, Baergen RN, Pellitteri PK, et al. Parathyroid lipoadenoma: case report and review of the literature. Otolaryngol Head Neck Surg 1996;114:313–6.

120. Ogrin C. A rare case of double parathyroid lipoadenoma with hyperparathyroidism. Am J Med Sci 2013;346:432–4.

121. Johnson N, Serpell JW, Johnson WR, et al. Parathyroid lipoadenoma. ANZ J Surg 2013. [Epub ahead of print].

122. Drickman A. Metastatic carcinoma involving the parathyroid glands. Report of two cases and a short review of the literature. Arch Surg 1961;82:576–8.

123. Fulciniti F, Pezzullo L, Chiofalo MG, et al. Metastatic breast carcinoma to parathyroid adenoma on fine needle cytology sample: report of a case. Diagn Cytopathol 2011;39(9):681–5.

124. Gattuso P, Khan NA, Jablokow VR, et al. Neoplasms metastatic to parathyroid glands. South Med J 1988;81:1467.

125. Lee HE, Kim DH, Cho YH, et al. Tumor-to-tumor metastasis: hepatocellular carcinoma metastatic to parathyroid adenoma. Pathol Int 2011;61:593–7.

126. Margolis CI, Goldenberg VE. Breast carcinoma metastatic to parathyroid adenoma. N Y State J Med 1969;69:702–3.

127. Venkatraman L, Kalangutkar A, Russell CF. Primary hyperparathyroidism and metastatic carcinoma within parathyroid gland. J Clin Pathol 2007;60:1058–60.

128. Liu F, Gnepp DR, Pisharodi LR. Fine needle aspiration of parathyroid lesions. Acta Cytol 2004;48:133–6.

129. Tseleni-Balafouta S, Gakiopoulou H, Kavantzas N, et al. Parathyroid proliferations: a source of diagnostic pitfalls in FNA of thyroid. Cancer 2007;111:130–6.

130. Tseng FY, Hsiao YL, Chang TC. Ultrasound-guided fine needle aspiration cytology of parathyroid lesions. A review of 72 cases. Acta Cytol 2002;46:1029–36.

131. Abati A, Skarulis MC, Shawker T, et al. Ultrasound-guided fine-needle aspiration of parathyroid lesions: a morphological and immunocytochemical approach. Hum Pathol 1995;26:338–43.

132. Grimelius L, Johansson H. Pathology of parathyroid tumors. Semin Surg Oncol 1997;13:142–54.

133. Portel-Gomes GM, Grimelius L, Johansson H, et al. Chromogranin A in human neuroendocrine tumors: an immunohistochemical study with region-specific antibodies. Am J Surg Pathol 2001;25:1261–7.

134. Khan A, Tischler AS, Patwardhan NA, et al. Calcitonin immunoreactivity in neoplastic and hyperplastic parathyroid glands: an immunohistochemical study. Endocr Pathol 2003;14:249–55.

135. McGregor DK, Khurana KK, Cao C, et al. Diagnosing primary and metastatic renal cell carcinoma: the use of the monoclonal antibody 'Renal Cell Carcinoma Marker'. Am J Surg Pathol 2001;25:1485–92.

136. Feng CC, Ding GX, Song NH, et al. Paraneoplastic hormones: parathyroid hormone-related protein (PTHrP) and erythropoietin (EPO) are related to vascular endothelial growth factor (VEGF) expression in clear cell renal cell carcinoma. Tumour Biol 2013;34(6):3471–6.

137. Porzionato A, Macchi V, Barzon L, et al. Immunohistochemical assessment of parafibromin in mouse and human tissues. J Anat 2006;209:817–27.

138. Cetani F, Ambrogini E, Viacava P, et al. Should parafibromin staining replace HRTP2 gene analysis as an additional tool for histologic diagnosis of parathyroid carcinoma? Eur J Endocrinol 2007;156:547–54.

139. Juhlin CC, Villablanca A, Sandelin K, et al. Parafibromin immunoreactivity: its use as an additional diagnostic marker for parathyroid tumor classification. Endocr Relat Cancer 2007;14:501–12.

140. Ozcan A, Shen SS, Hamilton C, et al. PAX 8 expression in non-neoplastic tissues, primary tumors, and metastatic tumors: a comprehensive immunohistochemical study. Mod Pathol 2011;24:751–64.

141. Canavese G, Azzoni C, Pizzi S, et al. p27: a potential main inhibitor of cell proliferation in digestive endocrine tumors but not a marker of benign behavior. Hum Pathol 2001;32:1094–101.

142. Perez-Martinez FC, Alonso V, Sarasa JL, et al. Immunohistochemical analysis of low-grade and high-grade prostate carcinoma: relative changes of parathyroid hormone-related protein and its parathyroid hormone 1 receptor, osteoprotegerin and receptor activator of nuclear factor-kB ligand. J Clin Pathol 2007;60:290–4.

143. Tominaga Y, Tsuzuki T, Uchida K, et al. Expression of PRAD1/cyclin D1, retinoblastoma gene

products, and Ki67 in parathyroid hyperplasia caused by chronic renal failure versus primary adenoma. Kidney Int 1999;55:1375–83.

144. Shattuck TM, Valimaki S, Obara T, et al. Somatic and germ-line mutations of the HRPT2 gene in sporadic parathyroid carcinoma. N Engl J Med 2003; 349:1722–9.

145. Cetani F, Pardi E, Borsari S, et al. Genetic analyses of the HRPT2 gene in primary hyperparathyroidism: germline and somatic mutations in familial and sporadic parathyroid tumors. J Clin Endocrinol Metab 2004;89:5583–91.

146. Krebs LJ, Shattuck TM, Arnold A. HRPT2 mutational analysis of typical sporadic parathyroid adenomas. J Clin Endocrinol Metab 2005;90:5015–7.

147. Niramitmahapanya S, Sunthornthepvarakul T, Deerochanawong C, et al. Sensitivity of HRPT2 mutation screening to detect parathyroid carcinoma and atypical parathyroid adenoma of Thai patients. J Med Assoc Thai 2011;94(Suppl 2):S17–22.

148. Cryns VL, Thor A, Xu HJ, et al. Loss of the retinoblastoma tumor-suppressor gene in parathyroid carcinoma. N Engl J Med 1994;330:757–61.

149. Pearce SH, Trump D, Wooding C, et al. Loss of heterozygosity studies at the retinoblastoma and breast cancer susceptibility (BRCA2) loci in pituitary, parathyroid, pancreatic and carcinoid tumours. Clin Endocrinol 1996;45:195–200.

150. Hendy GN, D'Souza-Li L, Yang B, et al. Mutations of the calcium-sensing receptor (CASR) in familial hypocalciuric hypercalcemia, neonatal severe hyperparathyroidism, and autosomal dominant hypocalcemia. Hum Mutat 2000;16:281–96.

151. D'Souza-Li L, Canaff L, Janicic N, et al. An acceptor splice site mutation in the calcium-sensing receptor (CASR) gene in familial hypocalciuric hypercalcemia and neonatal severe hyperparathyroidism. Hum Mutat 2001;18:411–21.

152. Chen RA, Goodman WG. Role of the calcium-sensing receptor in parathyroid gland physiology. Am J Phys 2004;286:F1005–11.

153. Skelly BJ, Franklin RJ. Mutations in genes causing human familial isolated hyperparathyroidism do not account for hyperparathyroidism in Keeshond dogs. Vet J 2007;174:652–4.

154. Juhlin CC, Nilsson IL, Johansson K, et al. Parafibromin and APC as screening markers for malignant potential in atypical parathyroid adenomas. Endocr Pathol 2010;21:166–77.

155. Svedlund J, Auren M, Sundstrom M, et al. Aberrant WNT/beta-catenin signaling in parathyroid carcinoma. Mol Cancer 2010;9:294.

156. Arnold A, Kim HG, Gaz RD, et al. Molecular cloning and chromosomal mapping of DNA rearranged with the parathyroid hormone gene in a parathyroid adenoma. Clin Investig 1989;83:2034–40.

157. Arnold A, Staunton CE, Kim HG, et al. Monoclonality and abnormal parathyroid hormone genes in parathyroid adenomas. N Engl J Med 1988;318: 658–62.

158. Cetani F, Pardi E, Giovannetti A, et al. Genetic analysis of the MEN1 gene and HPRT2 locus in two Italian kindreds with familial isolated hyperparathyroidism. Clin Endocrinol 2002;56:457–64.

159. Westin G, Bjorklund P, Akerstrom G. Molecular genetics of parathyroid disease. World J Surg 2009; 33:2224–33.

160. Sharretts JM, Simonds WF. Clinical and molecular genetics of parathyroid neoplasms. Best Pract Res Clin Endocrinol Metab 2010;24:491–502.

161. Chandrasekharappa SC, Guru SC, Manickam P, et al. Positional cloning of the gene for multiple endocrine neoplasia-type 1. Science 1997;276: 404–7.

162. Lemmens I, Van de Ven WJ, Kas K, et al. Identification of the multiple endocrine neoplasia type 1 (MEN1) gene. The European Consortium on MEN1. Hum Mol Genet 1997;6:1177–83.

163. Carrasco CA, Gonzalez AA, Carvajal CA, et al. Novel intronic mutation of MEN1 gene causing familial isolated primary hyperparathyroidism. J Clin Endocrinol Metab 2004;89:4124–9.

164. Cetani F, Pardi E, Ambrogini E, et al. Genetic analyses in familial isolated hyperparathyroidism: implication for clinical assessment and surgical management. Clin Endocrinol 2006;64:146–52.

165. Farnebo F, Teh BT, Dotzenrath C, et al. Differential loss of heterozygosity in familial, sporadic, and uremic hyperparathyroidism. Hum Genet 1997;99: 342–9.

166. Honda M, Tsukada T, Tanaka H, et al. A novel mutation of the MEN1 gene in a Japanese kindred with familial isolated primary hyperparathyroidism. Eur J Endocrinol 2000;142:138–43.

167. Howell VM, Cardinal JW, Richardson AL, et al. Rapid mutation screening for HRPT2 and MEN1 mutations associated with familial and sporadic primary hyperparathyroidism. J Mol Diagn 2006;8: 559–66.

168. Carling T, Correa P, Hessman O, et al. Parathyroid MEN1 gene mutations in relation to clinical characteristics of nonfamilial primary hyperparathyroidism. J Clin Endocrinol Metab 1998;83: 2960–3.

Assessing Biological Aggression in Adrenocortical Neoplasia

Isobel C. Mouat[a], Thomas J. Giordano, MD, PhD[a,b,c],*

KEYWORDS

- Adrenocortical neoplasia • Adrenocortical adenomas • Adrenocortical carcinomas
- Histologic grading • Molecular grading

ABSTRACT

Pathologists are highly skilled at the evaluation of adrenal neoplasms. Occasional adrenocortical tumors can be diagnostically challenging and supplementary tools can assist in these cases. Histologic and molecular studies support a model that includes 2 broad classes of adrenocortical carcinoma with distinct somatic genetic alterations and clinical outcomes. Pathologists should endeavor to grade adrenocortical carcinomas to assign each case into one of these 2 classes. Mitotic grading by mitotic counting and Ki-67 immunohistochemistry represent the most practicable and informative methods currently available.

OVERVIEW

The incidence of tumors of the adrenal cortex has steadily increased over the past few decades, largely due to increased use of clinical imaging studies. Fortunately, a vast majority of these incidentally discovered masses (so-called adrenal incidentalomas) are benign. Of these benign lesions, adrenocortical adenomas represent the most common pathologic entity. Conversely, adrenocortical carcinomas are rare tumors with malignant potential and an incidence of 1 to 2 cases per million.

When faced with the diagnostic challenge of an adrenal specimen with a mass, surgical pathologists must address several fundamental questions. First, broadly speaking, Is it a neoplasm? And, if so, What is the origin/differentiation of the neoplasm (ie, Is it a cortical or medullary tumor?)? Perhaps it is neither, such as a mesenchymal neoplasm or a metastasis. Second, once determining that a mass is of cortical origin, Does it possess malignant potential (ie, the ability to invade and metastasize)? If so, a diagnosis of carcinoma is appropriate. Alternatively, if the mass is cortical and lacks malignant potential, a diagnosis of adrenocortical adenoma should be rendered. In those cases of adrenocortical carcinoma, the remaining questions are related to stage and grade. Is the tumor confined to the adrenal gland (stages I and II) or is there extra-adrenal extension (stage III)? Finally, what is the biological aggression of the mass (ie, What is the grade of the neoplasm?)? Surgical pathologists have historically focused most of their attention on the first questions, What is the origin of the mass? Is it carcinoma? and What is the stage of disease? Increasing attention is being paid, however, to the final question of tumor grade and, by extension, determining what is the most informative grading method. This article briefly reviews the literature on these issues, with emphasis on histologic and molecular grading of adrenocortical carcinoma.

DIFFERENTIAL DIAGNOSIS OF ADRENAL MASSES

Compared with other organs, the differential diagnosis of the solitary adrenal mass is relatively

[a] Department of Pathology, University of Michigan Health System, Ann Arbor, MI, USA; [b] Department of Internal Medicine, University of Michigan Health System, Ann Arbor, MI, USA; [c] Comprehensive Cancer Center, University of Michigan Health System, Ann Arbor, MI, USA
* Corresponding author. Department of Pathology, University of Michigan Health System, 1150 West Medical Center Drive, MSRB1, 4520D, Ann Arbor, MI 48109-5602.
E-mail address: giordano@umich.edu

Surgical Pathology 7 (2014) 533–541
http://dx.doi.org/10.1016/j.path.2014.08.003

surgpath.theclinics.com

Key Features
OF ADRENOCORTICAL NEOPLASIA

Clinical, genetic, and radiologic

- Adrenocortical neoplasia can be hormonally functional or nonfunctional.

- Adrenocortical neoplasia is sporadic in most cases; syndromic forms are recognized (eg, Li-Fraumeni).

- Adrenocortical neoplasia is often incidentally discovered by imaging.

- Adenomas are often homogenous on imaging.

- Carcinomas are often heterogeneous with necrosis on imaging.

Gross pathology

- Adenomas tend to be small (<5 cm) and homogenous.

- Carcinomas tend to be large (>5 cm) with clonal nodularity and necrosis.

Histopathology for diagnosis

- Adenomas can be lipid rich, have a nested growth pattern, be low nuclear grade, have low mitotic counts, and lack invasion, necrosis, and atypical mitotic figures.

- Carcinoma are usually lipid poor, have a diffuse growth pattern, have high nuclear grade, have abundant mitoses, and display vascular invasion, necrosis, and atypical mitotic figures.

- There is immunoreactivity for α-inhibin, steroidogenesis factor (SF)-1, melan-A, and synaptophysin.

- Tumors are nonimmunoreactive for chromogranin and most keratins.

- Ki-67 index can be useful for diagnosis.

Histopathology for prognosis

- Mitotic grade defines 2 classes of carcinoma (low grade and high grade).

- Immunoreactivity for p53 and nuclear β–catenin supports a diagnosis of high-grade carcinoma.

- Ki-67 index can define prognostic subgroups of carcinoma.

Pitfalls
IN ASSESSMENT OF ADRENOCORTICAL NEOPLASIA

! Confusing cortical and medullary tumors

! Undersampling the capsule of a large cortical tumor, leading to an underappreciation of invasion

! Misinterpreting hemorrhage and organization in an adenoma as evidence of carcinoma

! Overdiagnosis of carcinoma based on large tumor size in the absence of supporting features of carcinoma

! Not grading carcinomas by mitotic counts and/or Ki-67 index

! Undergrading carcinoma diagnosed by needle biopsy

these diagnostic possibilities purely on histologic grounds. Occasional cases are challenging and for those cases a variety of diagnostic immunohistochemical tools are available.[1–3] In general,

Differential Diagnosis
OF ADRENOCORTICAL NEOPLASIA

Adrenocortical adenoma	Absence of Weiss parameters (invasion, high nuclear grade, mitoses, necrosis, and so forth); immunoprofile of a cortical tumor
Adrenocortical carcinoma	Presence of Weiss parameters (invasion, high nuclear grade, mitoses, necrosis, and so forth); immunoprofile of a cortical tumor
Medullary tumors	Nested growth pattern Amphophilic cytoplasm Chromogranin immunoreactivity
Miscellaneous primary tumors	Histopathology and immunprofile reflect the type of tumor
Adrenal metastases	Histopathology and immunprofile reflect the origin of the tumor

restricted. Adrenal masses are broadly divided into 4 categories: cortical, medullary, miscellaneous primary tumors, and metastases. Pathologists are highly skilled at differentiating between cortical tumors selectively express the following proteins, for which commercially established antibodies that robustly work with formalin-fixed paraffin-embedded tissues are available: α-inhibin,[4–7] SF-1,[1] melan-A,[8,9] and calretinin.[6,10] Expression of intermediate filaments is largely restricted to vimentin,[11] because cortical tumors poorly express most keratins despite being carcinomas.[12] Medullary tumors express S100 in a sustenacular pattern and diffusely express markers of neuroendocrine differentiation, such as chromogranin A.[13,14] Synaptophysin, a marker of neuroendocrine differentiation, is coexpressed in cortical and medullary neoplasms,[13] despite cortical tumors not being part of the neuroendocrine family of tumors.

Miscellaneous primary tumors and metastases have immunohistochemical profiles that reflect the specific type of tumor that is present. For example, leiomyomas of the adrenal gland express smooth muscle markers (eg, actins), angiosarcomas express vascular markers (eg, CD31), metastatic carcinomas express epithelial markers (keratins), and nonadrenal tissue-specific markers that reflect the organ of origin (eg, TTF1 expression in metastatic lung adenocarcinoma) and lymphomas express a variety of lymphoid markers depending on the lymphoma phenotype (eg, CD20). The combination of routine histologic assessment and immunohistochemistry, as needed for select cases, is highly effective in determining the type or origin of the vast majority of adrenal tumors.

ASSESSMENT OF MALIGNANT POTENTIAL IN ADRENOCORTICAL TUMORS BY ROUTINE HISTOLOGY AND IMMUNOHISTOCHEMISTRY

Once a pathologist has determined that a given adrenal tumor is of adrenocortical origin, the assessment of its malignant potential becomes paramount; this decision fundamentally determines the treatment plan. There was a time when pathologists found this differential diagnosis especially challenging and a certain level of mysticism surrounded the diagnosis of adrenocortical tumors. This situation was greatly impacted by 3 landmark studies that systematically examined multiple clinical and histologic features to derive characteristics associated specifically with malignant behavior.[15–17] Of these systematic studies, the Weiss system has obtained the widest acceptance by practicing pathologists,[18] largely a reflection of its ease of use. This system recently marked its 25th anniversary since its inception and has been incorporated into many molecular

studies.[19–22] Modifications designed to streamline the scoring parameters have been introduced[23,24] as well as similar systems for pediatric cases[25] and oncocytic tumors.[26,27] The main morphologic features of the Weiss system are illustrated in **Fig. 1**.

In addition, recent work has demonstrated that carcinomas have selective loss of their reticulin network compared with adenomas.[28,29] This knowledge provides another tool for the workup of adrenocortical neoplasms, allowing for additional corroboration of diagnosis.

Beyond these histologic assessments, a diagnostic role for the evaluation of the degree of tumor cell proliferation in adrenocortical tumors has emerged. Most such studies have focused on Ki-67 expression as assessed by MIB1 immunohistochemistry.[20,23,30–33] High expression of Ki-67 demonstrates high proliferative activity, thus supporting a diagnosis of adrenocortical carcinoma. Although no single immunohistochemical marker in isolation can distinguish adenoma and carcinoma in all cases, the Ki67 index adds value in a large majority of cases and has become a useful tool in the multifactorial evaluation of the separating adenomas and carcinomas (**Fig. 2**).

ASSESSMENT OF MALIGNANT POTENTIAL IN ADRENOCORTICAL TUMORS BY MOLECULAR METHODS

Adrenocortical neoplasms, despite their rare nature, have been extensively studied by a variety of molecular methods. Numerous individual molecular features have been investigated for their diagnostic potential as well as more recent comprehensive and genome-wide molecular characterizations. For example, individual markers shown to have utility in the diagnostic separation of adenoma and carcinoma include alteration of the of IGF2 locus, resulting in substantially increased expression in approximately 90% of adrenocortical carcinomas.[34] Looking back, the degree of progress has been remarkable. A complete review is beyond the scope of this article, but several recent reviews are available.[35–37]

One of the first genome-wide gene expression profiling studies of adrenocortical neoplasms came from the authors' laboratory and clearly showed that adenoma and carcinomas displayed profoundly distinct gene expression.[38] This study, although limited by a small number of tumors, clearly demonstrated the diagnostic potential of gene expression in adrenocortical tumors.

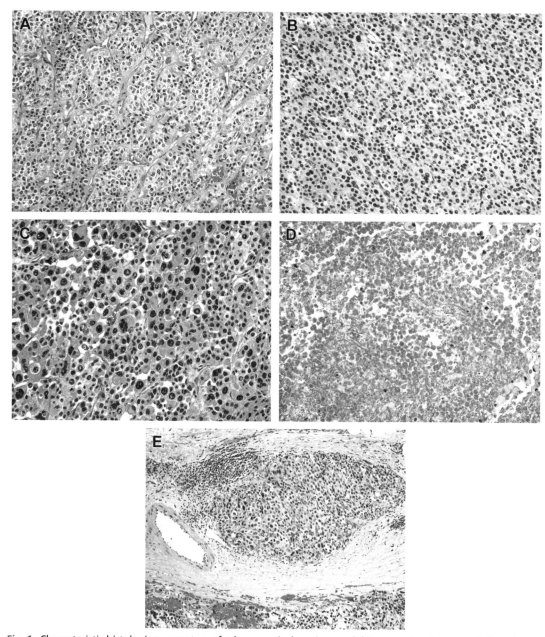

Fig. 1. Characteristic histologic parameters of adrenocortical carcinoma. (*A*) Low-grade adrenocortical carcinoma with nested growth pattern and low mitotic count. (*B*) Typical adrenocortical carcinoma with diffuse growth pattern and consisting of lipid-poor cells. (*C*) Adrenocortical carcinoma consisting of large cells with abundant lipid-poor eosinophilic cytoplasm and high-grade nuclei. (*D*) Adrenocortical carcinoma with coagulative tumor necrosis. (*E*) Adrenocortical carcinoma with angiolymphatic vascular invasion, with adjacent small artery. Hematoxylin-eosin, original magnification ×200.

Numerous similar studies confirmed and expanded these initial findings (reviewed by Assis and colleagues[39,40]). It is now accepted that adenomas and carcinomas have distinct gene expression profiles. The authors' group has attempted to distill these results into a molecular reverse transcription–polymerase chain reaction assay that can be used to confirm a diagnosis of carcinoma when needed and evaluate diagnostically difficult cases with equivocal features.[41]

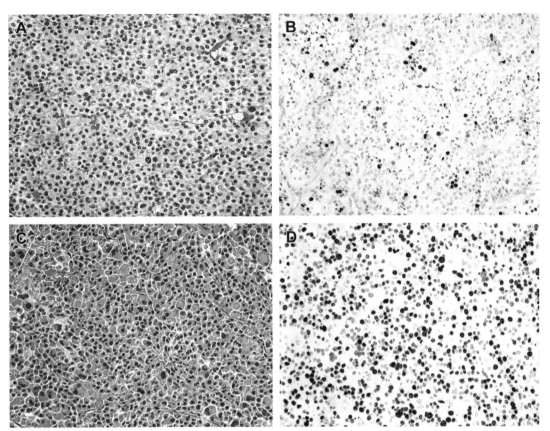

Fig. 2. Examples of low-grade and high-grade adrenocortical carcinomas with associated Ki-67 immunohisto-chemistry. (*A*) Low-grade adrenocortical carcinoma with rare mitotic figures. (*B*) Corresponding Ki-67 immunos-tain with a labeling index of approximately 10%. (*C*) High-grade adrenocortical carcinoma with mitotic figures. (*D*) Corresponding Ki-67 immunostain with a labeling index of approximately 80%. Original magnification ×200.

ASSESSMENT OF BIOLOGICAL AGGRESSION IN ADRENOCORTICAL CARCINOMAS BY ROUTINE HISTOLOGY AND IMMUNOHISTOCHEMISTRY

Once a diagnosis of adrenocortical carcinoma has been rendered, it is also the role of the pathologist to grade the carcinoma in an effort to predict its clinical course. This has been attempted using a variety of methods:

- Mitotic grade
- Stereoidogenic factor-1 (SF-1)
- Other proliferation-based scoring methods

MITOTIC GRADE

First, the Weiss score, as discussed previously, originally designed used to assess the malignant potential of a given tumor, also possesses prog-nostic significance[42]; high Weiss score tumors generally display aggressive clinical behaviors. In

the course of developing the Weiss system, Dr Weiss and colleagues noted that, among the indi-vidual Weiss parameters, mitotic count possessed the highest prognostic significance. This observa-tion led them to propose a 2-tier grading system based solely on mitotic rate. Low-grade carci-nomas were designated as having fewer than 20 mitoses per 50 high-power fields, whereas high-grade carcinomas had greater than 20 mitoses per 50 high-power fields. At the authors' center, this mitotic grading has become fully entrenched and essential to individualizing the treatment plan.[43,44] In the authors' opinion, mitotic grading of adrenocortical carcinoma is the gold standard against which other molecular grading methods must be judged, especially given the low cost of routine mitotic grading.

STEREOIDOGENIC FACTOR-1

Given its essential role in adrenal development,[45] there has been much interest in the expression of stereoidogenic factor-1 (SF-1) as a diagnostic and prognostic marker.[46,47] Validation studies confirm the expression of stereoidogenic factor 1 and reinforce its potential role as a prognostic marker, even in models that include Ki-67 index and mitotic count data.[48]

RELATED PROLIFERATION-BASED SCORING METHODS

Similar to its diagnostic role in separating adenoma and carcinoma, assessment of proliferation by alternative methods has been well studied. A recent article by Duregon and colleagues[49] compared 3 related methods for assessing proliferative activity in adrenocortical carcinoma: mitotic counts, phosphorhistone H3–specific immunohistochemistry, and Ki-67 expression by immunohistochemistry. The antibody against phosphohistone H3 targets the phosphorylated form of the H3 histone protein, which is preferentially detected during mitotic chromosome condensation.[50] Accordingly, immunohistochemical detection of phosphohistone H3 represents an alternative method for assessing the mitotic rate and has been deployed in studies of a wide range of tumor types, including other endocrine tumors.[51] In directly comparing these approaches in a cohort of 52 adrenocortical carcinomas using both manual and automated methods, they demonstrated that the Ki-67 index was the strongest predictor of overall survival. Moreover, they showed the Ki-67 index could divide the cases in 2 or 3 classes with significantly different survivals.

ASSESSMENT OF BIOLOGICAL AGGRESSION IN ADRENOCORTICAL CARCINOMAS BY MOLECULAR METHODS

Many studies have attempted to derive clinically meaningful classification schemes of adrenocortical carcinoma using molecular data. Among these, most have focused on genome-wide measurement of gene expression (ie, the transcriptome). Two such studies from independent groups (the European Network for the Study of Adrenal Tumors and the University of Michigan) divided adrenocortical carcinomas into 2 primary groups with distinctly different outcomes.[19,52]

In the case of the University of Michigan cohort, the subgroups reflected the mitotic grade. A gene expression derived measure, however, did provide incremental prognostic information in an outcome model that included tumor stage and mitotic grade, suggesting that gene expression data might yield a more refined grading.

Integration of information regarding the common somatic mutations observed in adrenocortical carcinoma provides a genetic framework for the 2-class model. Low- and high-grade tumors have approximately equal numbers of cases with altered IGF2 expression,[19,52] suggesting that alteration of the IGF2 locus with subsequent increase of IGF2 expression is an early event in adrenocortical carcinoma development. Conversely, somatic alterations of TP53 and CTNNB1 are enriched in high-grade adrenocortical carcinomas,[53] suggesting these mutations are late events in adrenocortical carcinoma development and may be defining alterations of high-grade tumors.[54] Beyond TP53 and CTNNB1, alterations of RB1 have been found associated with adrenocortical carcinomas with aggressive clinical behavior[55] and may represent an alternative path for the development of high-grade disease.

Other genomic technologies have been used to derive classification schemes of adrenocortical carcinoma, the results of which generally support a low- and high-grade model. Genome-wide assessment of copy number changes did reveal diagnostic significance and divided the carcinomas into 2 groups with distinct survival.[56] Similarly, DNA methylation studies have also divided adrenocortical carcinoma into 2 groups with distinct survival.[57] A recent integrated multiplatform genomic analysis confirmed 2 classes of adrenocortical carcinoma with distinct mutational profiles and clinical outcomes.[58]

ROUTINE GRADING OF ADRENOCORTICAL CARCINOMA

Given the consistent results from many studies that indicate adrenocortical carcinomas segregate into 2 groups with different clinical outcomes, it should become incumbent on pathologists to assign each case to an indolent (low-grade) or aggressive (high-grade) category. It remains to be determined exactly what is the most informative grading method that also can be easily deployed in all pathology laboratories, although recent studies suggest the Ki-67 index may be the most informative grading method.[49]

Once a diagnosis of adrenocortical has been rendered, mitotic grading by mitotic counting is required whenever sufficient tumor is available.[43] In cases of core biopsies where sampling errors are common, a tentative mitotic count and grade can be rendered along with a cautionary comment that the tumor grade might be higher than what is represented by the core biopsy.

Beyond mitotic counting, immunohistochemistry for Ki-67, p53, and β-catenin can be informative and these markers can be performed whenever tissue blocks are available. In particular, assessment of proliferation by Ki-67 can be useful when reviewing previously diagnosed cases in which there is a discrepancy between pathologists in mitotic counts. Suboptimal histologic preparations can make identification of mitotic figures difficult, resulting in discordant mitotic counts. In such cases, demonstration of a low or high Ki-67 labeling index can help resolve the discrepancy and thereby assist in accurate mitotic grading. Beyond diagnostically challenging cases, if the Ki-67 index is further shown the most informative prognostic biomarker, then this will quickly become the standard of care in addition to mitotic grade by mitotic counting.

Routine immunohistochemical assessment of p53 and β-catenin are a bit more controversial. On one hand, having strong nuclear staining for either of these markers suggests an underlying genetic mutation in TP53 or in one of the genes of the *wnt* pathway, usually CTNNB1. These findings are strongly associated with aggressive behavior[39] and support a diagnosis of high-grade adrenocortical carcinoma. On the other hand, knowledge of these results does not have a direct impact on the treatment plan; therefore, it has been argued that these stains do not provide independent data and lack medical value.

SUMMARY

Pathologists are highly skilled at the evaluation of adrenal neoplasms. Occasional adrenocortical tumors can be diagnostically challenging, however, and supplementary tools can assist in these cases. Histologic and molecular studies support a model that includes 2 broad classes of adrenocortical carcinoma with distinct somatic genetic alterations and clinical outcomes. Pathologists should endeavor to grade adrenocortical carcinomas to assign each case into one of these 2 classes. Mitotic grading by mitotic counting and Ki-67 immunohistochemistry represent the most practicable and informative methods currently available.

REFERENCES

1. Sasano H, Suzuki T, Moriya T. Recent advances in histopathology and immunohistochemistry of adrenocortical carcinoma. Endocr Pathol 2006;17: 345–54.

2. Mondal SK, Dasgupta S, Jain P, et al. Histopathological study of adrenocortical carcinoma with special reference to the Weiss system and TNM staging and the role of immunohistochemistry to differentiate it from renal cell carcinoma.

J Cancer Res Ther 2013;9:436–41. http://dx.doi.org/10.4103/0973-1482.119329.

3. Lapinski JE, Chen L, Zhou M. Distinguishing clear cell renal cell carcinoma, retroperitoneal paraganglioma, and adrenal cortical lesions on limited biopsy material: utility of immunohistochemical markers. Appl Immunohistochem Mol Morphol 2010;18:414–21. http://dx.doi.org/10.1097/PAI.0b013e3181ddf7b9.

4. Matias-Guiu X, Prat J. Alpha-inhibin immunostaining in diagnostic pathology. Adv Anat Pathol 1998;5:263–7.

5. Arola J, Liu J, Heikkila P, et al. Expression of inhibin alpha in the human adrenal gland and adrenocortical tumors. Endocr Res 1998;24:865–7.

6. Jorda M, De MB, Nadji M. Calretinin and inhibin are useful in separating adrenocortical neoplasms from pheochromocytomas. Appl Immunohistochem Mol Morphol 2002;10:67–70.

7. Fetsch PA, Powers CN, Zakowski MF, et al. Anti-alpha-inhibin: marker of choice for the consistent distinction between adrenocortical carcinoma and renal cell carcinoma in fine-needle aspiration. Cancer 1999;87:168–72.

8. Busam KJ, Iversen K, Coplan KA, et al. Immunoreactivity for A103, an antibody to melan-A (Mart-1), in adrenocortical and other steroid tumors. Am J Surg Pathol 1998;22:57–63.

9. Ghorab Z, Jorda M, Ganjei P, et al. Melan A (A103) is expressed in adrenocortical neoplasms but not in renal cell and hepatocellular carcinomas. Appl Immunohistochem Mol Morphol 2003;11:330–3.

10. Zhang H, Bu H, Chen H, et al. Comparison of immunohistochemical markers in the differential diagnosis of adrenocortical tumors: immunohistochemical analysis of adrenocortical tumors. Appl Immunohistochem Mol Morphol 2008;16:32–9. http://dx.doi.org/10.1097/PAI.0b013e318032cf56.

11. Henzen-Logmans SC, Stel HV, van Muijen GN, et al. Expression of intermediate filament proteins in adrenal cortex and related tumours. Histopathology 1988;12:359–72.

12. Gaffey MJ, Traweek ST, Mills SE, et al. Cytokeratin expression in adrenocortical neoplasia: an immunohistochemical and biochemical study with implications for the differential diagnosis of adrenocortical, hepatocellular, and renal cell carcinoma. Hum Pathol 1992;23:144–53.

13. Miettinen M. Neuroendocrine differentiation in adrenocortical carcinoma. New immunohistochemical findings supported by electron microscopy. Lab Invest 1992;66:169–74.

14. Schröder S, Padberg BC, Achilles E, et al. Immunocytochemistry in adrenocortical tumours: a clinicomorphological study of 72 neoplasms. Virchows Arch A Pathol Anat Histopathol 1992;420:65–70.

15. Hough AJ, Hollifield JW, Page DL, et al. Prognostic factors in adrenal cortical tumors. A mathematical

analysis of clinical and morphologic data. Am J Clin Pathol 1979;72:390–9.

16. Weiss LM. Comparative histologic study of 43 metastasizing and nonmetastasizing adrenocortical tumors. Am J Surg Pathol 1984;8:163–9.

17. van Slooten H, Schaberg A, Smeenk D, et al. Morphologic characteristics of benign and malignant adrenocortical tumors. Cancer 1985;55: 766–73.

18. Papotti M, Libè R, Duregon E, et al. The Weiss score and beyond–histopathology for adrenocortical carcinoma. Horm Cancer 2011;2:333–40. http://dx.doi.org/10.1007/s12672-011-0088-0.

19. de Reynies A, Assié G, Rickman DS, et al. Gene expression profiling reveals a new classification of adrenocortical tumors and identifies molecular predictors of malignancy and survival. J Clin Oncol 2009;27:1108–15. http://dx.doi.org/10.1200/JCO.2008.18.5678.

20. Schmitt A, Saremaslani P, Schmid S, et al. IGFII and MIB1 immunohistochemistry is helpful for the differentiation of benign from malignant adrenocortical tumours. Histopathology 2006;49:298–307. http://dx.doi.org/10.1111/j.1365-2559.2006.02505.x.

21. Gust L, Taieb D, Beliard A, et al. Preoperative 18F-FDG uptake is strongly correlated with malignancy, Weiss score, and molecular markers of aggressiveness in adrenal cortical tumors. World J Surg 2012;36:1406–10. http://dx.doi.org/10.1007/s00268-011-1374-2.

22. Duregon E, Rapa I, Votta A, et al. MicroRNA expression patterns in adrenocortical carcinoma variants and clinical pathologic correlations. Hum Pathol 2014;45(8):1555–62. http://dx.doi.org/10.1016/j.humpath.2014.04.005.

23. Aubert S, Wacrenier A, Leroy X, et al. Weiss system revisited: a clinicopathologic and immunohistochemical study of 49 adrenocortical tumors. Am J Surg Pathol 2002;26:1612–9.

24. Magro G, Esposito G, Cecchetto G, et al. Pediatric adrenocortical tumors: morphological diagnostic criteria and immunohistochemical expression of matrix metalloproteinase type 2 and human leucocyte-associated antigen (HLA) class II antigens. Results from the Italian Pediatric Rare Tumor (TREP) Study project. Hum Pathol 2012;43:31–9. http://dx.doi.org/10.1016/j.humpath.2011.04.016.

25. Wieneke JA, Thompson LD, Heffess CS. Adrenal cortical neoplasms in the pediatric population: a clinicopathologic and immunophenotypic analysis of 83 patients. Am J Surg Pathol 2003;27:867–81.

26. Bisceglia M, Ludovico O, Di Mattia A, et al. Adrenocortical oncocytic tumors: report of 10 cases and review of the literature. Int J Surg Pathol 2004;12: 231–43.

27. Wong DD, Spagnolo DV, Bisceglia M, et al. Oncocytic adrenocortical neoplasms–a clinicopathologic study of 13 new cases emphasizing the importance of their recognition. Hum Pathol 2011;42:489–99. http://dx.doi.org/10.1016/j.humpath.2010.08.010.

28. Volante M, Bollito E, Sperone P, et al. Clinicopathological study of a series of 92 adrenocortical carcinomas: from a proposal of simplified diagnostic algorithm to prognostic stratification. Histopathology 2009;55:535–43. http://dx.doi.org/10.1111/j.1365-2559.2009.03423.x.

29. Duregon E, Fassina A, Volante M, et al. The reticulin algorithm for adrenocortical tumor diagnosis: a multicentric validation study on 245 unpublished cases. Am J Surg Pathol 2013;37:1433–40. http://dx.doi.org/10.1097/PAS.0b013e31828d387b.

30. Vargas MP, Vargas HI, Kleiner DE, et al. The role of prognostic markers (MiB-1, RB, and bcl-2) in the diagnosis of parathyroid tumors. Mod Pathol 1997;10:12–7.

31. Babinska A, Sworczak K, Wisniewski P, et al. The role of immunohistochemistry in histopathological diagnostics of clinically "silent" incidentally detected adrenal masses. Exp Clin Endocrinol Diabetes 2008;116:246–51. http://dx.doi.org/10.1055/s-2007-993164.

32. Soon PS, Gill AJ, Benn DE, et al. Microarray gene expression and immunohistochemistry analyses of adrenocortical tumors identify IGF2 and Ki-67 as useful in differentiating carcinomas from adenomas. Endocr Relat Cancer 2009;16:573–83. http://dx.doi.org/10.1677/ERC-08-0237.

33. Morimoto R, Satoh F, Murakami O, et al. Immunohistochemistry of a proliferation marker Ki67/MIB1 in adrenocortical carcinomas: Ki67/MIB1 labeling index is a predictor for recurrence of adrenocortical carcinomas. Endocr J 2008;55:49–55.

34. Ribeiro TC, Latronico AC. Insulin-like growth factor system on adrenocortical tumorigenesis. Mol Cell Endocrinol 2012;351:96–100. http://dx.doi.org/10.1016/j.mce.2011.09.042.

35. Fassnacht M, Kroiss M, Allolio B. Update in adrenocortical carcinoma. J Clin Endocrinol Metab 2013;98:4551–64. http://dx.doi.org/10.1210/jc.2013-3020.

36. Bourdeau I, MacKenzie-Feder J, Lacroix A. Recent advances in adrenocortical carcinoma in adults. Curr Opin Endocrinol Diabetes Obes 2013;20:192–7. http://dx.doi.org/10.1097/MED.0b013e3283602274.

37. Else T, Kim AC, Sabolch A, et al. Adrenocortical carcinoma. Endocr Rev 2014;35:282–326. http://dx.doi.org/10.1210/er.2013-1029.

38. Giordano TJ, Thomas DG, Kuick R, et al. Distinct transcriptional profiles of adrenocortical tumors uncovered by DNA microarray analysis. Am J Pathol 2003;162:521–31. http://dx.doi.org/10.1016/S0002-9440(10)63846-1.

39. Assie G, Giordano TJ, Bertherat J. Gene expression profiling in adrenocortical neoplasia. Mol Cell

Endocrinol 2012;351:111–7. http://dx.doi.org/10.1016/j.mce.2011.09.044.

40. Assie G, Jouinot A, Bertherat J. The 'omics' of adrenocortical tumours for personalized medicine. Nat Rev Endocrinol 2014;10:215–28. http://dx.doi.org/10.1038/nrendo.2013.272.

41. Tomlins SA, Vinco M, Kuick R, et al. Development of a multi-gene qPCR assay for adrenocortical tumor diagnosis and prognosis. Mod Pathol 2013;26:138A.

42. van't Sant HP, Bouvy ND, Kazemier G, et al. The prognostic value of two different histopathological scoring systems for adrenocortical carcinomas. Histopathology 2007;51:239–45. http://dx.doi.org/10.1111/j.1365-2559.2007.02747.x.

43. Giordano TJ. The argument for mitotic rate-based grading for the prognostication of adrenocortical carcinoma. Am J Surg Pathol 2011;35:471–3. http://dx.doi.org/10.1097/PAS.0b013e31820bcf21.

44. Else T, Williams AR, Sabolch A, et al. Adjuvant therapies and patient and tumor characteristics associated with survival of adult patients with adrenocortical carcinoma. J Clin Endocrinol Metab 2014;99:455–61. http://dx.doi.org/10.1210/jc.2013-2856.

45. Gardiner JR, Shima Y, Morohashi K, et al. SF-1 expression during adrenal development and tumourigenesis. Mol Cell Endocrinol 2012;351:12–8. http://dx.doi.org/10.1016/j.mce.2011.10.007.

46. Sbiera S, Schmull S, Assie G, et al. High diagnostic and prognostic value of steroidogenic factor-1 expression in adrenal tumors. J Clin Endocrinol Metab 2010;95:E161–71. http://dx.doi.org/10.1210/jc.2010-0653.

47. Sangoi AR, Fujiwara M, West RB, et al. Immunohistochemical distinction of primary adrenal cortical lesions from metastatic clear cell renal cell carcinoma: a study of 248 cases. Am J Surg Pathol 2011;35:678–86. http://dx.doi.org/10.1097/PAS.0b013e3182152629.

48. Duregon E, Volante M, Giorcelli J, et al. Diagnostic and prognostic role of steroidogenic factor 1 in adrenocortical carcinoma: a validation study focusing on clinical and pathologic correlates. Hum Pathol 2013;44:822–8. http://dx.doi.org/10.1016/j.humpath.2012.07.025.

49. Duregon E, Molinaro L, Volante M, et al. Comparative diagnostic and prognostic performances of the hematoxylin-eosin and phospho-histone H3 mitotic count and Ki-67 index in adrenocortical

carcinoma. Mod Pathol 2014;27(9):1246–54. http://dx.doi.org/10.1038/modpathol.2013.230.

50. Juan G, Traganos F, James WM, et al. Histone H3 phosphorylation and expression of cyclins A and B1 measured in individual cells during their progression through G2 and mitosis. Cytometry 1998;32:71–7.

51. Draganova-Tacheva R, Bibbo M, Birbe R, et al. The potential value of phosphohistone-h3 mitotic index determined by digital image analysis in the assessment of pancreatic endocrine tumors in fine-needle aspiration cytology specimens. Acta cytol 2013;57:291–5. http://dx.doi.org/10.1159/000350885.

52. Giordano TJ, Kuick R, Else T, et al. Molecular classification and prognostication of adrenocortical tumors by transcriptome profiling. Clin Cancer Res 2009;15:668–76. http://dx.doi.org/10.1158/1078-0432.CCR-08-1067.

53. Ragazzon B, Libé R, Gaujoux S, et al. Transcriptome analysis reveals that p53 and {beta}-catenin alterations occur in a group of aggressive adrenocortical cancers. Cancer Res 2010;70:8276–81. http://dx.doi.org/10.1158/0008-5472.CAN-10-2014.

54. Kim A, Giordano TJ, Kuick R, et al. Wnt/betacatenin signaling in adrenocortical stem/progenitor cells: implications for adrenocortical carcinoma. Ann Endocrinol (Paris) 2009;70:156. http://dx.doi.org/10.1016/j.ando.2009.02.006.

55. Ragazzon B, Libé R, Assié G, et al. Mass-array screening of frequent mutations in cancers reveals RB1 alterations in aggressive adrenocortical carcinomas. Eur J Endocrinol 2014;170:385–91. http://dx.doi.org/10.1530/EJE-13-0778.

56. Barreau O, de Reynies A, Wilmot-Roussel H, et al. Clinical and pathophysiological implications of chromosomal alterations in adrenocortical tumors: an integrated genomic approach. J Clin Endocrinol Metab 2012;97:E301–11. http://dx.doi.org/10.1210/jc.2011-1588.

57. Barreau O, Assié G, Wilmot-Roussel H, et al. Identification of a CpG island methylator phenotype in adrenocortical carcinomas. J Clin Endocrinol Metab 2013;98:E174–84. http://dx.doi.org/10.1210/jc.2012-2993.

58. Assié G, Letouzé E, Fassnacht M, et al. Integrated genomic characterization of adrenocortical carcinoma. Nat Genet 2014;46:607–12. http://dx.doi.org/10.1038/ng.2953.

Paragangliomas Arising in the Head and Neck
A Morphologic Review and Genetic Update

Michelle D. Williams, MD[a],*, Thereasa A. Rich, MS[b]

KEYWORDS

- Paraganglioma ● SDHB immunohistochemistry ● Familial syndromes ● Morphology
- Head and neck neoplasms

ABSTRACT

Seventy percent of parasympathetic paragangliomas arise in the head and neck and are nonsecretory. Awareness of the differential diagnosis based on location, overlapping morphology, and immunohistochemical profiles aids in the correct diagnosis, particularly on limited tissue samples. Moreover, 30% to 40% of head and neck paragangliomas are known to be associated with hereditary syndromes, with the succinate dehydrogenase enzyme family comprising the most frequent association. The pathologist's role is becoming increasing critical for facilitating optimal patient care beyond the initial tissue diagnosis of paraganglioma to include screening and documenting potential hereditary tumors requiring further patient counseling and testing.

OVERVIEW

Paragangliomas (PGLs) are rare neuroendocrine neoplasms arising from the neuroectodermal crest associated with the sympathetic and parasympathetic nervous systems. The estimated incidence of extra-adrenal paragangliomas is 1 per 1 million persons. Compared with the sympathetic nervous system–derived PGLs, which arise predominately in the paraxial/prevertebral regions, including the organs of Zuckerkandl and extending into pelvic organs (ie, bladder), a majority of extra-adrenal paragangliomas (70%) arise in the head and neck region, specifically from the parasympathetic nervous system. Unlike the adrenal counterpart, pheochromocytoma (PHEO), which often secretes catecholamines (epinephrine and norepinephrine), a vast majority of head and neck PGLs are nonsecretory (>95%).[1,2]

The clinical presentation in the head and neck is often a painless neck mass arising in the 5th or 6th decade of life, although based on location, tinnitus and dysphagia may be reported. A majority of head and neck PGLs arise along the glossopharyngeal and vagus nerves, with the most common clinical sites the carotid artery bifurcation, middle ear, and jugular fossa (Fig. 1). Normal paraganglia are also present, however, in the supraglottic and infraglottic larynx and subclavian regions that also may also give rise to PGLs that are less frequently encountered and, therefore, may be more challenging to recognize secondary to the rarer location. PGLs have also been reported in the thyroid; parathyroid; orbit; and sinonasal region, including skull base, which, although rare, should be considered in the differential diagnosis of neuroendocrine tumors throughout the head and neck region.[1,3,4] Adding to the complexity of the anatomic locations is the clinical nomenclature of glomus, often associated with PGLs in the head and neck region, which may lead to confusion, because the term, *glomus*, pathologically refers to an unrelated pathologic entity. Other historic names included chemodactomas and nonchromaffin tumors.

ASSOCIATED GENETIC ALTERATIONS

Over the past 10 years, there has been an increasing focus on the genetic work-up of patients

Disclosure: The authors have no conflict of interest or any disclosures pertaining to this body of work.
[a] Department of Pathology, The University of Texas MD Anderson Cancer Center, 1515 Holcombe Boulevard, Unit 085, Houston, TX 77030, USA; [b] Clinical Cancer Genetics Program, The University of Texas MD Anderson Cancer Center, 1400 Hermann Pressler Drive, Unit 444, Houston, TX 77230, USA
* Corresponding author.
E-mail address: mdwillia@mdanderson.org

surgpath.theclinics.com

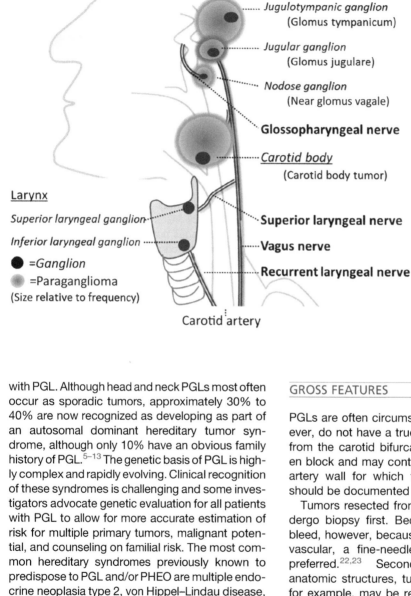

Middle ear
.... *Jugulotympanic ganglion*
    (Glomus tympanicum)

------------ *Jugular ganglion*
    (Glomus jugulare)

.... *Nodose ganglion*
    (Near glomus vagale)

Glossopharyngeal nerve

Carotid body
    (Carotid body tumor)

Larynx

Superior laryngeal ganglion········   **Superior laryngeal nerve**

Inferior laryngeal ganglion ··········   **Vagus nerve**

● =*Ganglion*   **Recurrent laryngeal nerve**
 =*Paraganglioma*
(Size relative to frequency)

Carotid artery

with PGL. Although head and neck PGLs most often occur as sporadic tumors, approximately 30% to 40% are now recognized as developing as part of an autosomal dominant hereditary tumor syndrome, although only 10% have an obvious family history of PGL.[5–13] The genetic basis of PGL is highly complex and rapidly evolving. Clinical recognition of these syndromes is challenging and some investigators advocate genetic evaluation for all patients with PGL to allow for more accurate estimation of risk for multiple primary tumors, malignant potential, and counseling on familial risk. The most common hereditary syndromes previously known to predispose to PGL and/or PHEO are multiple endocrine neoplasia type 2, von Hippel–Lindau disease, and neurofibromatosis type 1; however, familial PGL syndromes associated with succinate dehydrogenase (SDH) gene mutations are now recognized as the major cause of hereditary PGL in the head and neck region (**Table 1**).[7,9,14–21] The significance to pathologists is the availability of immunohistochemical (IHC) evaluation of SDH genes and how their expression pattern can screen for potential hereditary associated tumors.

GROSS FEATURES

PGLs are often circumscribed masses that, however, do not have a true capsule (**Fig. 2**). Tumors from the carotid bifurcation are usually removed en block and may contain portions of the carotid artery wall for which the presence and extent should be documented grossly.

Tumors resected from other locations may undergo biopsy first. Because core biopsies may bleed, however, because these lesions are highly vascular, a fine-needle aspiration approach is preferred.[22,23] Secondary to the complex anatomic structures, tumors of the tympanicum, for example, may be resected in pieces, leading to tissue distortion and less recognizable histologic features that trigger pattern recognition as PGL.

MICROSCOPIC FEATURES

Microscopically, PGLs demonstrate similar histologic features regardless of anatomic sight of origin. At low power, there is typically a nested

Table 1
Overview of clinical features of hereditary head and neck paraganglioma

Syndrome	Gene	Mean Proportion of All Head and Neck Paraganglioma[a,8,10,11,35,36]	Head and Neck Location	Other Locations	Multiple Pheochromocytoma/ Paraganglioma	Penetrance	Malignancy Risk
PGL1	SDHD	~23%	+++	+	>50%	~90%[b]	<10%
PGL4	SDHB	~12%	++	+++	~20%	30%–77%	~30%[c]
PGL3	SDHC	~4%	+++	+	~15%–20%	UNK	Low
PGL2	SDHAF2	UNK	+++	–	~90%	~100%[b]	–
PGL5	SDHA	UNK	+	+	Not reported	UNK	Low
N/A	TMEM127	UNK	+	+++ (PHEO)	~40%	UNK	<5%
N/A	MAX	UNK	–	+++ (PHEO)	~60%–70%	UNK	25%

Other genes associated with PHEO/PGL with fewer than 10 reported cases include KIF1B, EGLN1 (PHD2), HIF1A, and FH.

Abbreviations: –, not reported; +, reported rarely; ++, occasional; +++, frequent; N/A, not assigned; UNK, unknown; PHEO, pheochromocytoma.

[a] Pooled estimate from references.

[b] When mutation in inherited paternally.

[c] Overall malignancy rate for SDHB PGL for all sites (including abdomen); specific rate for head and neck sites still to be defined.

Adapted from Refs.[19–21]

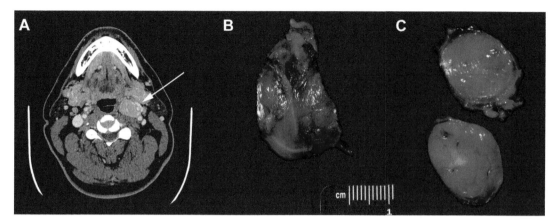

Fig. 2. Carotid body PGL. (*A*) CT evaluation of an expansile mass in the carotid bifurcation (*arrow*); (*B*) gross resection specimen showing circumscription; and (*C*) homogeneous cut surface.

proliferation of tumor cells surrounded by thin delicate fibrovascular septa known as the *zellenballen pattern* (**Fig. 3**). The edge of these lesions may show extension into adjacent soft tissue, or into the vascular wall, which should be documented, although this does not alter the diagnosis or predict malignancy. The tumor cells may range from round to polygonal or plasmacytoid, with some cases showing oncocytic, spindled, and lipid cell degeneration leading to clear morphology

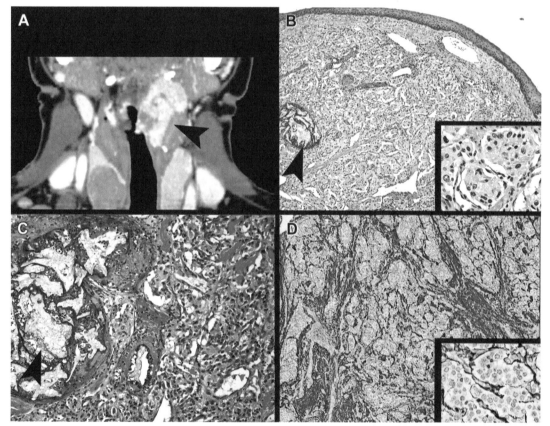

Fig. 3. Laryngeal (supraglottic) PGL. (*A*) CT scan of large supraglottic mass (*arrow*); (*B*) low power of submucal nested proliferation with overlying mucosa, embolization material (*arrow*), high-power (*inset ×200*) (hematoxylin and eosin, original magnification ×40); (*C*) higher-power of embolization material (*arrow*) with associated inflammatory reaction (hematoxylin and eosin, original magnification ×100); and (*D*) reticilin stain highlights the nested zellenballen growth pattern, high-power (*inset ×200*) (original magnification ×40).

(Fig. 4). Varying degrees of hyalinization and sclerosis distort the classic nested pattern (Fig. 5).

At higher power, the cells may be homogeneous with round hyperchromatic to salt-and-pepper nuclei with condensed chromatin and prominent nucleoli. Nuclear atypia may be present and marked either de novo as endocrine atypia or secondary to prior surgical embolization. Nuclear atypia does not have diagnostic significance in PGLs of the head and neck. Presurgical embolization is common and histologic changes associated with this prior treatment should be recognized and not confused with malignant changes. Embolization may lead to tumor necrosis, marked inflammatory infiltration obscuring the background neuroendocrine process, and resulting fibrosis, also distorting the typical nested visual pattern. Patients may have also undergone prior radiation to stabilize growing lesions, which also contribute to cytologic atypia and fibrosis in these lesions.

Additional features that should be documented in the pathology report include any invasive growth pattern into the blood vessel wall or adjacent tissue, the presence and extent of necrosis (may occur postembolization), and the presence and quantitation of mitoses.[24,25] While these features should be included in pathologic reporting of PGL, no hematoxylin-eosin (H&E) staining morphologic feature alone can predict biologic behavior and the term, *malignant*, should not be used outside of documented lymph node or distant metastases.

VARIANTS OF PARAGANGLIOMA

Because a vast majority of PGLs show classic morphologic features, variants, including sclerosing and pigmented PGLs, require awareness of these subtypes to avoid misclassifying as a malignant tumor. In the sclerosing variant of PGL, marked collagenous stroma distorts the nests of tumor cells and may lead to small clusters to single cells, poorly visualized in the sclerotic areas. The vascular network is also lost or distorted visually, although in the majority of cases reported by Plaza and

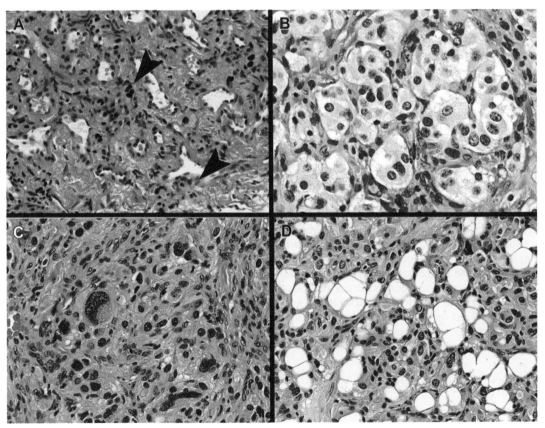

Fig. 4. Variations in microscopic features of PGL (*A*) prominent vasculature mimicking hemangioma showing scattered intervening paraganglia cells (*arrows*) (hematoxylin and eosin, original magnification ×200); (*B*) enlarged paraganglia cells with ample cytoplasm, round nuclei with prominent nucleoli, and condensed, clumped chromatin (hematoxylin and eosin, original magnification ×400); (*C*) prominent nuclear atypia with bizarre forms and spindled forms (right side) (hematoxylin and eosin, original magnification ×400); and (*D*) clearing within a PGL secondary to adipophillic metaplasia (hematoxylin and eosin, original magnification ×400).

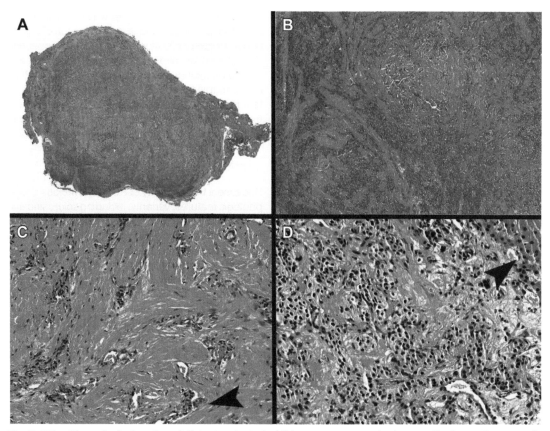

Fig. 5. PGL with marked sclerosis and distant metastasis. (*A*) Low-power vaguely circumscribed mass (hematoxylin and eosin, original magnification ×10); (*B*) dense sclerosis distorting nested pattern (hematoxylin and eosin, original magnification ×20); (*C*) marked vasculature, with scant compressed PGL cells (*arrow*) (hematoxylin and eosin, original magnification ×100); and (*D*) corresponding metatastatic PGL retaining a nested, bland growth pattern in the liver (*arrow*) in a core biopsy (hematoxylin and eosin, original magnification ×100).

colleagues,[26] at least a focal conventional nested pattern was identified within each tumor leading to the morphologic consideration of PGL. Pigmented extra-adrenal PGL is a rarely encountered variant in which the prominent intracytoplasmic pigment may obscure the nuclear/neuroendocrine features.[27] Because pigmentation may also rarely be present in other neuroendocrine tumors (neuroendocrine carcinoma, olfactory neuroblastoma, and medullary thyroid carcinoma), awareness and immunophenotypic support are needed combined with anatomic location for proper classification.

DIFFERENTIAL DIAGNOSIS

The differential diagnosis in the head and neck region requires consideration of the site of the lesion in combination with the histologic features identified in the biopsy or resection specimen, with differential diagnoses for neck masses, larynx, middle ear and, sinonasal, skull base specifically addressed in **Table 2**. Neuroendocrine tumors should be considered in the differential diagnosis in all regions of the head and neck when the morphology is not classic for a specific entity or neuroendocrine features are noted. Additionally, variants of PGL, in particular the sclerosing variant of PGL, need to be differentiated from other malignant infiltrating carcinomas and, including neuroendocrine carcinoma, and medullary thyroid carcinoma based on location.[26] Additionally, PGLs with pigmentation lead to a differential diagnosis, including melanoma.[27]

NECK MASSES

Because carotid body tumors are the most commonly encountered head and neck PGLs and they arise in a vary specific anatomic location, tumors arising outside of the classic area of the carotid bifurcation should raise concern of a lesion mimicking a PGL. Metastases to the neck from medullary thyroid carcinoma, Merkel cell carcinoma, and large or small cell carcinoma of the lung or other sites all have neuroendocrine cytologic features; however, they often show high-grade cytologic features and lack of nested growth pattern and express cytokeratin on IHC evaluation (**Fig. 6**). Because a neck mass may be the initial presentation of these diseases as an unknown primary, careful morphologic and IHC evaluation aid in the correct classification. Tumors with prominent clear cell change lead to the added differential of metastatic renal cell carcinoma, which may also overlap morphologically secondary to the prominent vascularization, nesting, and clearing.

LARYNX

PGLs are normally present in the supraglottic and infraglottic larynx and may give rise to PGLs in this region (see **Fig. 3**); however, because this is an uncommon site of origin and critical anatomic location, a surgical biopsy is often performed for initial evaluation. Biopsy tissue of the submucosal mass often shows the nested zellenballen pattern, which, however, may be distorted or crushed, limiting morphologic classification. The main differential in this region is with neuroendocrine carcinoma/atypical carcinoids, which also may arise in the supraglottic larynx, solid adenoid cystic, and basaloid squamous carcinoma (see **Fig. 6**). Usually, the solid growth pattern, lack of nesting, and associated vasculature, with higher-grade nuclear features, including mitoses, allows for differentiation. Immunohisothemical evaluation is also valuable on small biopsies for differentiation. Because atypical carcinoids may have an aggressive course, differentiating these entities pathologically is required.

IMMUNOHISTOCHEMICAL EVALUATION/ PROFILE

A diagnosis of PGL is made combining the morphologic features, clinical location (when classic), and, as appropriate, IHC evaluation to support lineage (**Fig. 7**). The paraganglia cells are negative for cytokeratins, which are a key marker to differentiate this entity from known malignant entities in the differential diagnosis (carcinoids, middle ear adenoma, medullary thyroid carcinoma, large cell neuroendocrine carcinoma, and Merkel cell carcinoma). Synaptophysin and chromogranin are both positive in a majority of PGLs regardless of site of origin and help support neurocrest origin (see **Fig. 3**A), whereas meningioma and metastatic renal cell carcinoma are negative for these markers.

Although S100 can be used to highlight supportive sustentacular cells, caution to not mistake reticulated S100 positive dendritic cells, which may be present in a range of processes, as sustentacular cells, is advised. The PGL cells are S100 negative (see **Fig. 3**B).

A determination of benign versus potentially malignant PGL cannot be made by H&E evaluation alone and using the term, malignant, in the pathologic report requires documented metastases to lymph nodes or distant sites. IHC evaluation, however, of the PGL cells for SDHB expression may (1) aid in determining risk of malignant potential and (2) assist in identifying PGL that may be hereditary, having an impact on both a patient's further follow-up/surveillance and potentially on identifying a family members' risk for PGLs.

Immunohistochemical Evaluation for Succinate Dehydrogenase Alterations

There is growing evidence IHC evaluation for SDHB has strong utility in detecting patients likely to carry a germline mutation in any of the genes of the SDH family, including SDHA, SDHB, SDHC, or SDHD.[28–31] In normal tissues, the SDHB protein shows a characteristic cytoplasmic IHC staining pattern in the cytoplasm corresponding to its mitochondrial location (see **Fig. 3**C). Because the SDH family of proteins (A, B, C, and D) bind together to form the mitochondrial complex II anchored to the inner mitochondrial membrane, alterations in any of the 4 genes (A, B, C or D) disrupts the overall complex formation/function. The SDHB IHC antibody is sensitive to the complex alteration and thus staining is lost if any of the 4 SDH family members is mutated. In all 128 PGL tumors studied to date from patients with a confirmed germline mutation of SDHA, SDHB, SDHD, or SDHC, loss of SDHB staining has been observed.[29–31]

In practice, SDHB IHC evaluation of PGLs in the head and neck may show loss in 30% to 40% of cases, which is added diagnostic information for advising genetic counseling and testing. Evaluation of SDHB IHC expression and the determination of loss of expression in PGL cells mandate the presence of a positive control in every case (**Box 1**, see **Fig. 3**D). The prevalent vasculature within PGL shows positive staining in the endothelial cells and thus should be identified in every case as positivity staining prior to an interpretation of the PGL as negative (SDHB expression loss). Additionally, as background, add-mixed inflammatory cells also retain SDHB staining, careful review to determine if the tumor cells are negative is also warranted. Reporting results must take into account that SDHB IHC is a screening process for the SDH family of genes' status (intact vs mutated) and that loss of SDHB IHC correlates with a germline condition; however, genetic counseling and further testing to determine which gene loci may

Table 2
Differential diagnoses of paragangliomas in the head and neck based on site of origin

| Differential Diagnosis by Site | Key Histologic Features | | Immunohistochemistry | | | Associations |
	Morphologic Features	Nuclear Features	Keratin	Chromogranin	S100	Familial Syndromes
Paraganglioma (PGL)	Circumscribed (no capsule), nested growth, scant stroma, prominent vasculature (variants sclerotic, pigmented), ample cytoplasm	Round with clumped chromatin; nucleoli; variable pleomorphism; no/low proliferation	–	+	–(+S cells only)	See Table 1 and MEN2, VHL, NF1
DDX for neck						Overlapping with PGLs
Medullary thyroid carcinoma	Infiltrative, nested, or solid	Variable cytoplasm	+	+	–	MEN2
Neuroendocrine carcinoma (large or small cell, Merkle carcinoma)	Infiltrative, solid, ± necrosis	Scant cytoplasm, hyperchromatic, frequent mitoses, ± nucleoli	+	+	–	NF1, VHL
Metastatic renal cell carcinoma	Circumscribed, scant stroma,	Nucleoli, lacking chromatin clumping, may mitoses	+	–	–	VHL, SDH
DDX for middle ear						
Meningioma	Whirls, lobulated, maybe clear	Dispersed chromatin, inconspicuous nucleoli	–(+EMA)	–	±	
Hemangioma	Vessel prominent with intervening stroma, cellularity between vessels not present	Bland with dispersed chromatin	–	–	–	
Middle ear adenoma	Non-nested, glandular, absence of prominent vascularity	Indistinct cell borders, round fine granular, no nucleoli	+	±	±	
Also consider renal cell carcinoma if clear						

DDX for larynx					
Solid adenoid cystic carcinoma	Infiltrative, no delicate vessels, solid (non-nested)	Hyperchromatic, scant cytoplasm, inconspicuous nucleoli	+	–	–
Basaloid squamous carcinoma	Infiltrative, desmoplasia, necrosis	Hyperchromatic, scant cytoplasm,	+	–	–
Neuroendocrine carcinoma (atypical carcinoid)	Infiltrative, solid or nested	Round to oval with clumped chromatin; ±nucleoli; low-grade is monotonous	+	+	–
DDX for sinonasal skull base					
Olfactory neuroblastoma (esthesioneuroblastoma)	Lobular, possible rosettes and background neurofilament, scant cytoplasm	Round with clumped chromatin; ±nucleoli; low-grade is monotonous	–	–	–(+S cells only)
Sinonasal-type hemangiopericytoma (glomangiopericytoma)	Cellularity between vessels not nested, more likely spindled cells	Monotonous cells, round, even chromatin, no/low proliferation	–	–	–
Melanoma	Poorly circumscribed, non-nested, no vascular network	Variable cytology, ±prominent nucleoli	–(Rarely +)	–	Usually +
Pituitary adenoma or ectopic	Nested, monomorphous	Round nuclei, inconspicuous nucleoli	+	±	Rare+
Also consider hemangioma and menigioma					

Abbreviations: DDX, differential diagnosis; EMA, epithelial membrane antigen; MEN2, multiple endocrine neoplasia type 2; NF1, neurofibromatosis type 1; S cells, sustentacular cells; SDH, succinate dehydrogenase; VHL, von Hippel-Lindau; +, positive; –, negative.

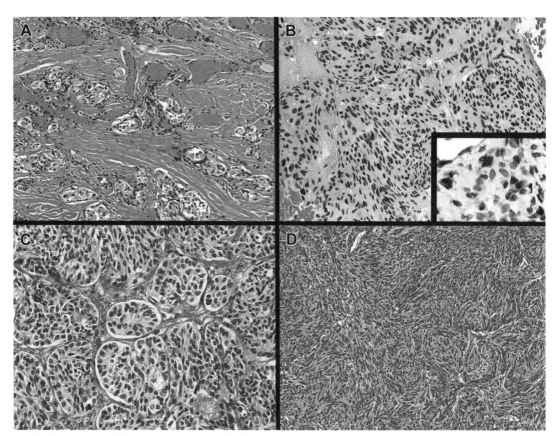

Fig. 6. Morphologic differential diagnosis. (*A*) PGL with dense hyalinized stroma splaying the tumor nests. The vasculature is not apparent (hematoxylin and eosin, original magnification ×40). (*B*) Metastatic PGL to skull base mimicking olfactory neuroblastoma; loss of SDHB by IHC aided in the diagnosis (*inset ×400*) (hematoxylin and eosin, original magnification ×100). (*C*) Nested medullary thyroid carcinoma in lymph node presenting as an unknown primary in the neck (hematoxylin and eosin, original magnification ×100). (*D*) Neuroendocrine carcinoma (atypical carcinoid) in the supraglottic larynx also showing a nested growth pattern (hematoxylin and eosin, original magnification ×100).

be involved are advised and critical to determine a PGL's malignant potential (see **Table 1**).

Furthermore, it has been shown that in addition to loss of SDHB staining, SDHA staining is possible and is also lost in patients with germline SDHA mutations.[28] In contrast to SDHB, the SDHA specific antibody is lost only when SDHA is mutated and expression is retained whether other SDH family members are altered or not.[28] It is hypothesized that SDHC and SDHD protein staining would also be negative in patients with a corresponding germline mutation; however, this has not been systematically studied and commercial antibodies are not yet available.[32] Pathologists, therefore, have an increasing role in supplementing the genetic evaluation of patients with PGL, analogous to the use of microsatellite instability testing and immunostaining for mismatch repair proteins in the identification of patients with Lynch syndrome.[33]

With the recognition of these critical clinicopathologic correlations, a recent consensus for reporting extra-adrenal PGL includes both details of IHC SDH evaluation and specific emphasis for the clinical information to be documented with each case.[24]

PROGNOSIS

The prognosis of patients with sporadic head and neck PGLs in general is favorable because a majority are indolent/benign and typically slow growing. Although complete resection is curative, because tumors are not encapsulated and in difficult anatomic locations, follow-up is still generally advised. Additionally, because there is a high risk of cranial nerve damage based on the tumor location, resection is not always advisable, leading to a small portion of head and neck PGLs receiving external beam radiation to stabilize growing tumors. The outcome in patients with the familial PGL syndromes continues to be defined because patients may develop multiple tumors leading to

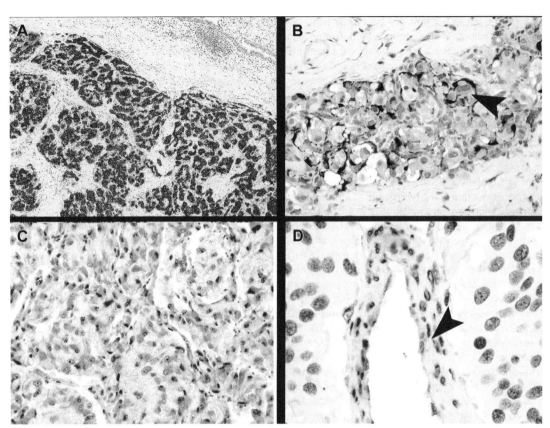

Fig. 7. IHC evaluation of PGL. (*A*) Chromogranin positivity (original magnification ×40); (*B*) paraganglia cells are negative for S100 (*arrow*) cuffed by supporting S100-positive sustentacular cells (original magnification ×200); (*C*) normal SDHB positivity in all cells (paraganglia, endothelial, and inflammatory cells) (original magnification ×200); and (*D*) SDHB negative paraganglia cells. SDHB positivity in the endothelial cells (internal control, *arrow*). Confirmed case of germline mutation in SDH (original magnification ×400).

additional comorbidities base on location and number of PGLs that develop. Malignant potential in head and neck PGLs overall remains low, less than 10% overall, although directly influenced by the underlying associated gene alterations (see **Table 1**).

HEREDITARY: FAMILIAL PARAGANGLIOMA SYNDROMES (SUCCINATE DEHYDROGENASE ENZYME GENES)

The most common hereditary form of head and neck PGLs is familial PGL syndrome type 1 (PGL1), accounting for 12.7% to 38.5% of all cases of head and neck PGLs, followed by (PGL4) types 4 (5%–27.3% of head and neck PGL) and 3 (PGL3) (0%–4.3% of head and neck PGL).[8,10,11,34,35] These syndromes result from inactivating germline mutations in the SDHD, SDHB, and SDHC genes, which encode subunits D, B, and C of the mitochondrial complex II SDH enzyme, respectively.[36–38] Patients with hereditary PGL syndromes are typically diagnosed at younger ages than their SDH-negative counterparts (mean 36.2 years vs 50.2 years) and more often have multiple tumors (46% vs 5%).[10] PGL1 is associated primarily with parasympathetic

---

Box 1
Pitfalls in evaluation of paraganglioma for succinate dehydrogenase, subunit B, expression by immunohistochemistry (IHC)

SDHB IHC

1. Must have positive internal control to evaluate for tumor loss of expression (ie, endothelial cells).

2. Beware of inflammatory and endothelial cell positivity admixed with negative PGL cells.

3. Reporting SDHB IHC expression loss by IHC indicates that genetic testing and counseling are advised.

4. Reporting SDHB IHC loss does not indicate which SDH gene may be altered (ie, A, B, C, or D).

head and neck PGLs that are frequently bilateral/multifocal, although sympathetic PGLs may also occur.[7,9,18,35,39–42] It is a highly penetrant syndrome but only when inherited from an individual's father, and malignant PGL is estimated to occur in fewer than 10%.[42]

SDHB gene mutations more often cause sympathetic PGLs arising within the abdomen, pelvis, or thorax but may also occur in the head and neck and are particularly associated with high risk for malignancy.[7,9,11,12,35,39,40,42] The higher malignancy risk relative to SDHB mutation carriers might be a consequence of the typical site of tumor development being the abdomen. It is not completely clear whether head and neck tumors in SDHB mutation carriers have higher rates of malignant transformation than head and neck tumors in SDHD mutation carriers. Nonetheless, germline mutations in SDHB are one of the most important predictors of risk for malignant PGL in general, occurring in 30% of tumors that arise in patients with this mutation, and an underlying germline mutation in SDHB is responsible for approximately half of all cases of malignant PGL.[5,6] Genetic testing for SDHB mutations should be considered for all patients with malignant PGL and those with elevated concern for malignancy because many patients who ultimately are found with malignant PHEO/PGL do not have evidence of metastases at initial diagnosis.[7] SDHB is associated with reduced penetrance of PGL (estimated at up to 30% by age 70), so are more likely to present as a single tumor with negative family history than SDHD mutation carriers.[7,9]

SDHC mutations are rare, responsible for only approximately 3% to 4% of head and neck PGLs, even though these are the predominant tumor in the syndrome.[8,10,34,35] Similar to SDHB, many SDHC mutation carriers present with a single tumor and apparently negative family history, also suggesting reduced penetrance of PGLs.

SDH mutations are also associated with gastrointestinal stromal tumors (GISTs) and renal tumors, and there is recent growing evidence that they are also associated with pituitary tumors.[43–48] Thus, SDHB IHC evaluation would also show findings similar to PGL in these tumors.[49] The association of PGL and GIST is also referred to as the Carney-Stratakis dyad or Carney-Stratakis syndrome, not to be confused with the Carney triad, which is the nonfamilial association of PGL, GIST, and pulmonary chondroma.[50]

SDHB, SDHD, and SHDC mutations are transmitted in an autosomal dominant manner, and additionally, SDHD mutations are associated with parent of origin effects. An SDHD mutation carrier still has a 50% risk to pass the mutation to each child (regardless of the gender of the parent or child); however, only individuals who inherit an SDHD mutation from their father have a high risk for PGL development.

Mutations in SDHAF2 (also known as SDH5) cause hereditary PGL syndrome type 2 and seems to be a rare cause of PGL given that they have only been identified in 2 families.[51,52] To date, SDHAF2 has been exclusively associated with head and neck PGLs and have a high probability of occurring bilaterally.

OTHER GENES ASSOCIATED WITH PARAGANGLIOMAS

Several other genes (SDHA, MAX, TMEM127, KIF1B, EGLN1 [PHD2], HIF2A, and FH) have more recently been connected with risk for PHEO/PGL; however, much less is known about the range of phenotypic expression given how few mutation carriers have been reported.[53–58] PGL syndrome type 5 (caused by mutations in SDHA) has only been described in a handful of cases and seems to confer low-penetrance susceptibility to PHEO, PGL, GIST, and possibly pituitary tumors. Most of the described mutation carriers have had a nonfamilial/apparently sporadic presentation. To date, all affected MAX mutation carriers have developed PHEO first, with some going on to develop an additional PGL, but no cases of head and neck PGLs have been described. TMEM127 has primarily been associated with PHEO rather than PGL and is frequently bilateral. Only 1 case of head and neck PGL has been described in a TMEM127 mutation carrier.[58] Only 1 case of PHEO in a KIF1B mutation carrier has been described. Inherited or postzygotic PHD2 and HIF2A mutations have been reported recently in a few patients with congenital polycythemia and either PHEO or PGL.[59–61] Germline mutations in FH, the gene responsible for autosomal dominant hereditary leiomyomatosis and renal cell cancer (HLRCC) and autosomal recessive fumarase deficiency, were recently reported in 5 cases of PHEO or PGL (including 1 patient with a carotid body PGL), who did not have classic features of HLRCC.[62] PHEO/PGL associated with FH mutations seem to have a higher rate of malignancy.

Complicated genetic testing algorithms that take into account tumor location, multifocality, biochemical phenotype, and presence of malignancy have been proposed that can help prioritize genetic tests needed, to reduce cost.[17,56,63] It is likely that next-generation sequencing technologies will be increasingly used, because they may be more cost effective to sequence all genes of interest simultaneously rather than in a stepwise fashion, particularly given the large degree of clinical overlap between syndromes. Moreover, as ancillary tools become available, as with SDH antibodies for immunohiotochemical evaluation of PGLs, the pathologist's role becomes increasing critical for facilitating optimal patient care through documentation of markers indicating potential hereditary tumors.

REFERENCES

1. DeLellis RA, Lloyd RV, Heitz PU, et al. Pathology and genetics of tumours of endocrine organs. Lyon (France): IARC Press; 2004.
2. Forbes JA, Brock AA, Ghiassi M, et al. Jugulotympanic paragangliomas: 75 years of evolution in understanding. Neurosurg Focus 2012;33(2):E13. http://dx.doi.org/10.3171/2012.6.FOCUS12138.
3. Yu BH, Sheng WQ, Wang J. Primary paraganglioma of thyroid gland: a clinicopathologic and immunohistochemical analysis of three cases with a review of the literature. Head Neck Pathol 2013;7(4):373–80. http://dx.doi.org/10.1007/s12105-013-0467-7.
4. Levy MT, Braun JT, Pennant M, et al. Primary paraganglioma of the parathyroid: a case report and clinicopathologic review [review]. Head Neck Pathol 2010;4(1):37–43. http://dx.doi.org/10.1007/s12105-009-0157-7.
5. Neumann HP, Bausch B, McWhinney SR, et al. Germ-line mutations in nonsyndromic pheochromocytoma. N Engl J Med 2002;346:1459–66.
6. Amar L, Bertherat J, Baudin E, et al. Genetic testing in pheochromocytoma or functional paraganglioma. J Clin Oncol 2005;23:8812–8.
7. Neumann HP, Pawlu C, Peczkowska M, et al. Distinct clinical features of paraganglioma syndromes associated with SDHB and SDHD gene mutations. JAMA 2004;292:943–51.
8. Schiavi F, Boedeker CC, Bausch B, et al. Predictors and prevalence of paraganglioma syndrome associated with mutations of the SDHC gene. JAMA 2005;294:2057–63.
9. Ricketts CJ, Forman JR, Rattenberry E, et al. Tumor risks and genotype-phenotype-proteotype analysis in 358 patients with germline mutations in SDHB and SDHD. Hum Mutat 2010;31:41–51.
10. Burnichon N, Rohmer V, Amar L, et al. The succinate dehydrogenase genetic testing in a large prospective series of patients with paragangliomas. J Clin Endocrinol Metab 2009;94:2817–27.
11. Jafri M, Whitworth J, Rattenberry E, et al. Evaluation of SDHB, SDHD and VHL gene susceptibility testing in the assessment of individuals with non-syndromic phaeochromocytoma, paraganglioma and head and neck paraganglioma. Clin Endocrinol (Oxf) 2013;78:898–906.
12. Boedeker CC, Neumann HP, Maier W, et al. Malignant head and neck paragangliomas in SDHB mutation carriers. Otolaryngol Head Neck Surg 2007;137:126–9.
13. Klein RD, Jin L, Rumilla K, et al. Germline SDHB mutations are common in patients with apparently sporadic sympathetic paragangliomas. Diagn Mol Pathol 2008;17:94–100.
14. Brandi ML, Gagel RF, Angeli A, et al. Guidelines for diagnosis and therapy of MEN type 1 and type 2. J Clin Endocrinol Metab 2001;86:5658–71.
15. Lonser RR, Glenn GM, Walther M, et al. von Hippel-Lindau disease. Lancet 2003;361:2059–67.
16. Hersh JH. Health supervision for children with neurofibromatosis. Pediatrics 2008;121:633–42.
17. Waguespack SG, Rich T, Grubbs E, et al. A current review of the etiology, diagnosis, and treatment of pediatric pheochromocytoma and paraganglioma. J Clin Endocrinol Metab 2010;95:2023–37.
18. Pasini B, Stratakis CA. SDH mutations in tumorigenesis and inherited endocrine tumours: lesson from the phaeochromocytoma-paraganglioma syndromes. J Intern Med 2009;266:19–42.
19. Boedeker CC, Hensen EF, Neumann HP, et al. Genetics of hereditary head and neck paragangliomas. Head Neck 2014;36(6):907–16.
20. Welander J, Soderkvist P, Gimm O. Genetics and clinical characteristics of hereditary pheochromocytomas and paragangliomas. Endocr Relat Cancer 2011;18:R253–76.
21. Kirmani S, Young WF. Hereditary paraganglioma-pheochromocytoma syndromes. In: Pagon RA, Adam MP, Bird TD, et al, editors. Seattle (WA): GeneReviews; 1993.
22. Fleming MV, Oertel YC, Rodríguez ER, et al. Fine-needle aspiration of six carotid body paragangliomas. Diagn Cytopathol 1993;9(5):510–5.
23. Rana RS, Dey P, Das A. Fine needle aspiration (FNA) cytology of extra-adrenal paragangliomas. Cytopathology 1997;8(2):108–13.
24. Mete O, Tischler AS, de Krijger R, et al. Protocol for the examination of specimens from patients with pheochromocytomas and extra-adrenal paragangliomas. Arch Pathol Lab Med 2014;138(2):182–8. http://dx.doi.org/10.5858/arpa.2012-0551-OA.
25. Lack EE, Lloyd RV, Carney JA, et al, Association of Directors of Anatomic and Surgical Pathology. Recommendations for the reporting of extra-adrenal paragangliomas. The Association of Directors of Anatomic and Surgical Pathology. Hum Pathol 2003;34(2):112–3.
26. Plaza JA, Wakely PE Jr, Moran C, et al. Sclerosing paraganglioma: report of 19 cases of an unusual variant of neuroendocrine tumor that may be mistaken for an aggressive malignant neoplasm. Am J Surg Pathol 2006;30(1):7–12.

27. Moran CA, Albores-Saavedra J, Wenig BM, et al. Pigmented extraadrenal paragangliomas. A clinicopathologic and immunohistochemical study of five cases. Cancer 1997;79(2):398–402.

28. Korpershoek E, Favier J, Gaal J, et al. SDHA immunohistochemistry detects germline SDHA gene mutations in apparently sporadic paragangliomas and pheochromocytomas. J Clin Endocrinol Metab 2011;96:E1472–6.

29. Gill AJ, Benn DE, Chou A, et al. Immunohistochemistry for SDHB triages genetic testing of SDHB, SDHC, and SDHD in paraganglioma-pheochromocytoma syndromes. Hum Pathol 2010;41:805–14.

30. van Nederveen FH, Gaal J, Favier J, et al. An immunohistochemical procedure to detect patients with paraganglioma and phaeochromocytoma with germline SDHB, SDHC, or SDHD gene mutations: a retrospective and prospective analysis. Lancet Oncol 2009;10:764–71.

31. Castelblanco E, Santacana M, Valls J, et al. Usefulness of negative and weak-diffuse pattern of SDHB immunostaining in assessment of SDH mutations in paragangliomas and pheochromocytomas. Endocr Pathol 2013;24:199–205.

32. Eisenhofer G, Tischler AS, de Krijger RR. Diagnostic tests and biomarkers for pheochromocytoma and extra-adrenal paraganglioma: from routine laboratory methods to disease stratification. Endocr Pathol 2012;23:4–14.

33. Umar A, Boland CR, Terdiman JP, et al. Revised Bethesda guidelines for hereditary nonpolyposis colorectal cancer (Lynch syndrome) and microsatellite instability. J Natl Cancer Inst 2004;96:261–8.

34. Baysal BE, Willett-Brozick JE, Lawrence EC, et al. Prevalence of SDHB, SDHC, and SDHD germline mutations in clinic patients with head and neck paragangliomas. J Med Genet 2002;39:178–83.

35. Neumann HP, Erlic Z, Boedeker CC, et al. Clinical predictors for germline mutations in head and neck paraganglioma patients: cost reduction strategy in genetic diagnostic process as fall-out. Cancer Res 2009;69:3650–6.

36. Baysal BE, Ferrell RE, Willett-Brozick JE, et al. Mutations in SDHD, a mitochondrial complex II gene, in hereditary paraganglioma. Science 2000;287:848–51.

37. Niemann S, Muller U. Mutations in SDHC cause autosomal dominant paraganglioma, type 3. Nat Genet 2000;26:268–70.

38. Astuti D, Latif F, Dallol A, et al. Gene mutations in the succinate dehydrogenase subunit SDHB cause susceptibility to familial pheochromocytoma and to familial paraganglioma. Am J Hum Genet 2001;69:49–54.

39. Timmers HJ, Gimenez-Roqueplo AP, Mannelli M, et al. Clinical aspects of SDHx-related pheochromocytoma and paraganglioma. Endocr Relat Cancer 2009;16:391–400.

40. Benn DE, Gimenez-Roqueplo AP, Reilly JR, et al. Clinical presentation and penetrance of pheochromocytoma/paraganglioma syndromes. J Clin Endocrinol Metab 2006;91:827–36.

41. Schiavi F, Dematte S, Cecchini ME, et al. The endemic paraganglioma syndrome type 1: origin, spread, and clinical expression. J Clin Endocrinol Metab 2012;97:E637–41.

42. van Hulsteijn LT, Dekkers OM, Hes FJ, et al. Risk of malignant paraganglioma in SDHB-mutation and SDHD-mutation carriers: a systematic review and meta-analysis. J Med Genet 2012;49:768–76.

43. Ayala-Ramirez M, Feng L, Johnson MM, et al. Clinical risk factors for malignancy and overall survival in patients with pheochromocytomas and sympathetic paragangliomas: primary tumor size and primary tumor location as prognostic indicators. J Clin Endocrinol Metab 2011;96:717–25.

44. Malinoc A, Sullivan M, Wiech T, et al. Biallelic inactivation of the SDHC gene in renal carcinoma associated with paraganglioma syndrome type 3. Endocr Relat Cancer 2012;19:283–90.

45. Ricketts C, Woodward ER, Killick P, et al. Germline SDHB mutations and familial renal cell carcinoma. J Natl Cancer Inst 2008;100:1260–2.

46. Pasini B, McWhinney SR, Bei T, et al. Clinical and molecular genetics of patients with the Carney-Stratakis syndrome and germline mutations of the genes coding for the succinate dehydrogenase subunits SDHB, SDHC, and SDHD. Eur J Hum Genet 2008;16:79–88.

47. Papathomas TG, Gaal J, Corssmit EP, et al. Non-pheochromocytoma (PCC)/paraganglioma (PGL) tumors in patients with succinate dehydrogenase-related PCC-PGL syndromes: a clinicopathological and molecular analysis. Eur J Endocrinol 2014;170:1–12.

48. Xekouki P, Pacak K, Almeida M, et al. Succinate dehydrogenase (SDH) D subunit (SDHD) inactivation in a growth-hormone-producing pituitary tumor: a new association for SDH? J Clin Endocrinol Metab 2012;97:E357–66.

49. Gill AJ, Chou A, Vilain R, et al. Immunohistochemistry for SDHB divides gastrointestinal stromal tumors (GISTs) into 2 distinct types. Am J Surg Pathol 2010;34:636–44.

50. Stratakis CA, Carney JA. The triad of paragangliomas, gastric stromal tumours and pulmonary chondromas (Carney triad), and the dyad of paragangliomas and gastric stromal sarcomas (Carney-Stratakis syndrome): molecular genetics and clinical implications. J Intern Med 2009;266:43–52.

51. Hao HX, Khalimonchuk O, Schraders M, et al. SDH5, a gene required for flavination of succinate

dehydrogenase, is mutated in paraganglioma. Science 2009;325:1139–42.

52. Bayley JP, Kunst HP, Cascon A, et al. SDHAF2 mutations in familial and sporadic paraganglioma and phaeochromocytoma. Lancet Oncol 2010;11: 366–72.

53. Burnichon N, Briere JJ, Libe R, et al. SDHA is a tumor suppressor gene causing paraganglioma. Hum Mol Genet 2010;19:3011–20.

54. Mason EF, Sadow PM, Wagner AJ, et al. Identification of succinate dehydrogenase-deficient bladder paragangliomas. Am J Surg Pathol 2013;37: 1612–8.

55. Dwight T, Mann K, Benn DE, et al. Familial SDHA mutation associated with pituitary adenoma and pheochromocytoma/paraganglioma. J Clin Endocrinol Metab 2013;98:E1103–8.

56. Peczkowska M, Kowalska A, Sygut J, et al. Testing new susceptibility genes in the cohort of apparently sporadic phaeochromocytoma/paraganglioma patients with clinical characteristics of hereditary syndromes. Clin Endocrinol (Oxf) 2013;79(6):817–23.

57. Yao L, Schiavi F, Cascon A, et al. Spectrum and prevalence of FP/TMEM127 gene mutations in pheochromocytomas and paragangliomas. JAMA 2010;304:2611–9.

58. Neumann HP, Sullivan M, Winter A, et al. Germline mutations of the TMEM127 gene in patients with paraganglioma of head and neck and extraadrenal abdominal sites. J Clin Endocrinol Metab 2011;96: E1279–82.

59. Eltzschig HK, Eckle T, Grenz A. PHD2 mutation and congenital erythrocytosis with paraganglioma. N Engl J Med 2009;360:1361–2 [author reply: 1362].

60. Ladroue C, Carcenac R, Leporrier M, et al. PHD2 mutation and congenital erythrocytosis with paraganglioma. N Engl J Med 2008;359:2685–92.

61. Zhuang Z, Yang C, Lorenzo F, et al. Somatic HIF2A gain-of-function mutations in paraganglioma with polycythemia. N Engl J Med 2012;367:922–30.

62. Castro-Vega LJ, Buffet A, de Cubas AA, et al. Germline mutations in FH confer predisposition to malignant pheochromocytomas and paragangliomas. Hum Mol Genet 2014;23(9):2440–6.

63. Erlic Z, Rybicki L, Peczkowska M, et al. Clinical predictors and algorithm for the genetic diagnosis of pheochromocytoma patients. Clin Cancer Res 2009;15:6378–85.

Pancreatic Neuroendocrine Neoplasms

J.N. Rosenbaum, MD, Ricardo Vincent Lloyd, MD, PhD*

KEYWORDS

- Pan-NEN • Pancreas • Neuroendocrine • Cancer • Ki-67 • Insulinoma • Glucagonoma
- Gastrinoma

ABSTRACT

Pancreatic neuroendocrine neoplasms (Pan-NENs) are rare but clinically important lesions. Pan-NENs are known for and often categorized by their capacity to produce clinical syndromes mediated by the production of hormones. Despite sometimes presenting dramatically from excessive hormone production, not all Pan-NENs produce functional hormone, and they can pose diagnostic challenges to practicing pathologists. Distinguishing Pan-NENs from mimics can be crucial, because Pan-NENs carry different prognoses and have unique treatments available due to their specific biological properties. This article reviews the current categorization and features of Pan-NENs.

***Typical Histologic Features*
OF PAN-NEN**

Architecture – multiple architectural types can coexist

- Solid (most common) – A/I
- Gyriform – B/II
- Glandular – C/III
- Undifferentiated – D/IV

Cytology

- Small, uniform, cuboidal cells
- Usually rounded or polygonal
- Finely granular cytoplasm (neurosecretory granules)
- Generally low mitotic rate
- Pleomorphism can be marked, but does not impact grade or stage

Nuclear features

- Central nuclei
- Coarse "salt and pepper" heterochromatin
- Nucleoli variably present

OVERVIEW

Pan-NENs are rare but clinically significant.[1–3] Pan-NENs are often categorized by their capacity to produce clinical syndromes mediated by the production of hormones. Despite sometimes presenting dramatically, not all Pan-NENs produce functional hormone, and they can present diagnostic challenges to clinicians and practicing pathologists. Distinguishing Pan-NEN from potential mimics can be crucial, because Pan-NENs often carry different prognoses and have unique treatments available due to their specific biological properties.

Historically, the nomenclature applied to tumors arising out of the neuroendocrine tissue of the pancreas has been diverse and often difficult to use in the daily practice of pathology. Currently, the terms, *pancreatic neuroendocrine neoplasm* and *pancreatic neuroendocrine tumor*, are preferred.[4,5] Such terminology unifies Pan-NENs with gastrointestinal neuroendocrine neoplasms

Disclosure Statement: The authors have nothing to disclose.
Department of Surgical Pathology, University of Wisconsin Hospital and Clinics, Room A4/204-3224, 600 Highland Ave., Madison, WI 53792-3224, USA
* Corresponding author. Pathology and Laboratory Medicine, University of Wisconsin School of Medicine and Public Health, 600 Highland Drive, Madison, WI 53792.
E-mail address: rvlloyd@wisc.edu

Surgical Pathology 7 (2014) 559–575
http://dx.doi.org/10.1016/j.path.2014.08.005

(GI-NENs), or carcinoids. These lesions share a common histologic appearance and often have similar clinical behavior (including paraneoplastic hormonal syndromes). The term, *islet cell tumor*, is to be avoided; these tumors can transdifferentiate and express hormone not produced by normal islets, and some of these lesions may originate from multipotent ductal (rather than islet) precursors. The terms, *carcinoma* and *adenoma*, are also problematic, because they imply a prognosis that current techniques are currently unable to determine.[2]

CLINICAL AND RADIOGRAPHIC FINDINGS

Pan-NEN is an uncommon pancreatic lesion, constituting approximately 1% to 2% of pancreatic neoplasms. Because of the capacity of Pan-NENs to produce functional hormone, these neoplasms can have dramatic clinical presentations. Although some subtypes (discussed later) show gender predilection, overall, men and women are affected in approximately equal proportion. They can arise at any age but are most common between the fourth and sixth decades. Pan-NENs, in particular nonfunctional subtypes, can follow an indolent course. On autopsy, studies find that between 1% and 5% of pancreata contain a clinically silent (and usually small) Pan-NEN as an incidental finding.[6]

Symptoms due to Pan-NEN generally fall into 2 categories: obstructive symptoms and hormonal syndromes. Obstructive symptoms are often vague, including abdominal pain, early satiety, decreased appetite, biliary obstruction, and sometimes a palpable mass.[3,6,7] Syndromic effects vary with tumor subtype and are discussed later. Generally, whether or not functional hormone is produced by a neoplasm is unrelated to its size.[3,7] It is true, however, that functional lesions tend to come to clinical attention sooner and are, therefore, smaller at the time of presentation and diagnosis.

Pan-NENs can vary substantially in size, with most between 1 and 5 cm, although some lesions can reach 20 cm or greater. Lesions less than 0.5 cm are classified as microadenomas. In general, larger lesions are associated with a greater risk of malignancy. As discussed previously, functional lesions most often present at smaller sizes, usually less than 2 cm in diameter. Pan-NEN is usually a solitary lesion. Multifocal disease should always raise the possibility of an underlying genetic syndrome, in particular multiple endocrine neoplasia, type 1 (MEN1).

RADIOLOGY

Evaluation of Pan-NENs is largely the domain of pathologists, because the grading and staging criteria can only be truly determined histologically.

Key features of pancreatic neuroendocrine neoplasms			
	Clinical Syndromic Features	Special Histologic Features	Preferred Treatment
Insulinoma	Whipple triad of hyperinsulinemic hypoglycemia	Amyloid	Total or subtotal pancreatectomy
Glucagonoma	Necrolytic migratory erythema		Subtotal pancreatectomy; octreotide
Gastrinoma	Zollinger-Ellison syndrome of multiple severe gastric and duodenal ulcers	Multiple neoplasms involving duodenal wall	Gastrectomy, tumor excision if resectable; octreotide, proton pump inhibitors
Somatostatinoma	Diabetes mellitus, cholelithiasis, weight loss, steatorrhea, diarrhea	Psammoma calcification	Total or subtotal pancreatectomy; octreotide
VIPoma	Watery diarrhea		Total or subtotal pancreatectomy; octreotide
Serotoninoma	Carcinoid—watery diarrhea with flushing	Argentaffinity	
Nonfunctional	Obstructive symptoms	Immunohistochemistry (IHC) can be positive for hormone, despite lack of clinical symptoms	Total or subtotal pancreatectomy

Pitfalls
IN THE DIAGNOSIS OF PANCREATIC NEUROENDOCRINE NEOPLASMS

! Gastric ulcer—multiple pancreatic tumors negative for gastrin, with gastrinomas actually OUTSIDE pancreas (often in the duodenum)

! In the setting of chronic pancreatitis, proliferating islet cells can be confused with Pan-NEN.

! Entrapped non-neoplastic ducts can lead to mistaken diagnosis of mixed endocrine/ductal carcinoma.[40]

! Clear cell change in of von Hippel-Lindau disease (VHL) can be confused with metastatic renal cell carcinoma (RCC).

! Hyperinsulinemic hypoglycemia is not exclusively caused by insulinoma (insulinlike growth factor [IGF]-2 release from solitary fibrous tumors and hypersecretion of insulin in nesidioblastosis).

! Reactive changes in nondysplastic islets in the context of functional Pan-NENs or postresection Pan-NENs.

! Vasoactive intestinal polypeptide (VIP) hypersecretion can be due to ganglioneuroma (more common in children).

! Metastatic squamous cell carcinoma (SCC) of the lung can be difficult to distinguish from primary SCC of the pancreas by histology alone.

Radiologic evaluation of Pan-NENs still plays an important role, however, especially in a patient's initial workup and surgical planning.[8–10] Ultrasound (US) can aid in diagnosis of Pan-NENs, although the modality is more typically part of a workup for obstructive symptoms. On US, Pan-NENs are round or oval, well-circumscribed hypoechoic masses. CT and MRI are the radiographic modalities of choice in a suspected pancreatic neoplasm, providing greater fields of view and resolution. CT or MRI can visualize calcifications, which are much more prevalent in Pan-NENs (20%) than in pancreatic adenocarcinoma (2%). Typically, Pan-NENs are isodense and vascular; however, larger, nonfunctional lesions can exhibit cystic degeneration or necrosis.

Somatostatin Scintigraphy (Octreotide Scan) and Functional Imaging

Somatostatin receptors (SSRTs) allow neuroendocrine neoplasms (NENs) to be targeted for radiology or radiotherapy.[8–12] The technique, of course, requires the presence of functional SSRTs

on the lesion of interest (discussed later). Overall, the technique has a sensitivity estimated at 80% to 90% for detection of NENs. Based primarily on the prevalence of receptors, sensitivity is highest for gastrinoma and lowest for primary insulinoma. The use of SSRT scintigraphy is currently of limited utility in nonmalignant insulinoma, although it can be effective in malignant disease.

Stimulation of pancreatic endocrine tumors with bioactive molecules (such as secretin or calcium) in a technique known as provocative angiography can help reveal cryptic neoplasms.[1,8] The technique involves administering the molecule sequentially to specific arteries and subsequently sampling the hepatic vein for products released secondary to the stimulation. The levels of the product molecules after each stimulus can reveal the arterial supply of a cryptic neoplasm. Secretin stimulates the release of gastrin from G-cell neoplasms, whereas calcium is a nonspecific secretagogue. Because β-cell neoplasms can be difficult to detect by SSRT scintigraphy or other means, provocative angiography is most useful in this context.

GROSS PATHOLOGY

Pan-NENs are usually solitary, discrete masses (**Fig. 1A**). Fibrosis can be significant, giving the lesion a firm consistency with a white to yellow color. More cellular lesions often have more of a pink caste, sometimes reminiscent of ectopic spleen.[1] Calcifications can occasionally be observed grossly or radiologically. Cystic or hemorrhagic changes can accompany larger lesions.[13,14]

HISTOPATHOLOGY

Four architectural types or patterns have been identified, historically. These are categorized as A–D or I–IV and are not pathognomonic of any subtype but can be helpful. A majority of lesions of any subclassification are type A/I with a solid architecture (**Fig. 2A**). β-Cell or α-cell neoplasms tend to exhibit type B/II gyriform architecture (see **Fig. 1B**), whereas G-cell neoplasms and VIPomas show type C/III glandular architecture. Type D/IV, or nondescript, architecture encompasses poorly differentiated or undifferentiated lesions. Multiple architectural types can be seen in the same lesion (**Fig. 3**).[3]

As with other GI-NENs, Pan-NENs are composed of small, relatively uniform, cuboidal cells containing central nuclei (compare **Figs. 1B** and **2A**; **Fig. 4A**). The cells are usually rounded or polygonal but can also conform to the overall architectural pattern (see **Fig. 3**). For example, a

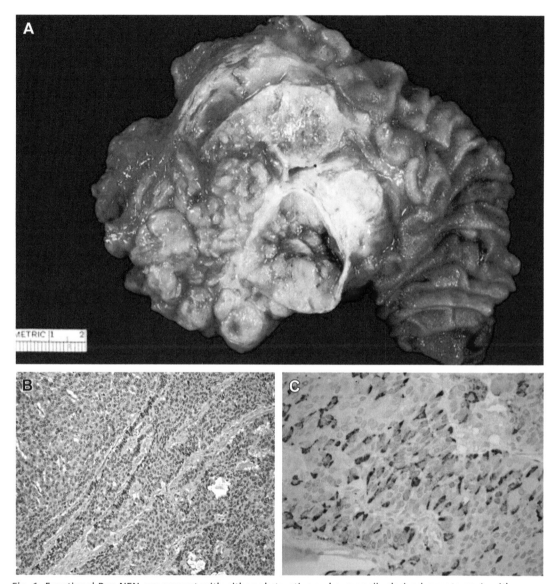

Fig. 1. Functional Pan-NEN can present with either obstructive or hormonally derived symptoms. In either case, the standard treatment of Pan-NEN is surgical resection of the pancreas, total or in part. Grossly, the Whipple resection specimen reveals the tumor in the head of the pancreas adjacent to the duodenum (*A*). A representative section of the tumor stained with hematoxylin-eosin (×10) shows infiltrating tumor cells (*B*). IHC for glucagon (*C*) identifies the tumor as Pan-NEN of α-cell origin (glucagonoma, ×40).

neoplasm with elongate, gyriform architecture may have cells that are also elongate.[2] The nuclei often (although not always) exhibit the coarsely granular heterochromatin, which lends a salt-and-pepper appearance to the nuclei. Nuclear enlargement and atypia can be marked,[15] and nucleoli are variably present. Neurosecretory granules give the cytoplasm a finely granular appearance, a feature that can be a useful diagnostic aid. The granules are argyrophilic and visible on electron microscopy, providing assistance in distinguishing difficult cases; however, it should be kept in mind that the undifferentiated neoplasms may not exhibit secretory granules at all.

Periodic acid–Schiff (PAS) staining can reveal positively staining globules of α_1-antitrypsin, either intra- or extracellularly, but detection of glycogen is usually minimal. Trapped normal glandular structures can occur and can themselves trap or produce extracellular mucus. Foamy cytoplasm, indicating an excess of lipid, may be observed.[16] This phenomenon is not usually associated with β-cell neoplasms. Clear cell change can be seen, particularly in the context of VHL (**Fig. 5** and

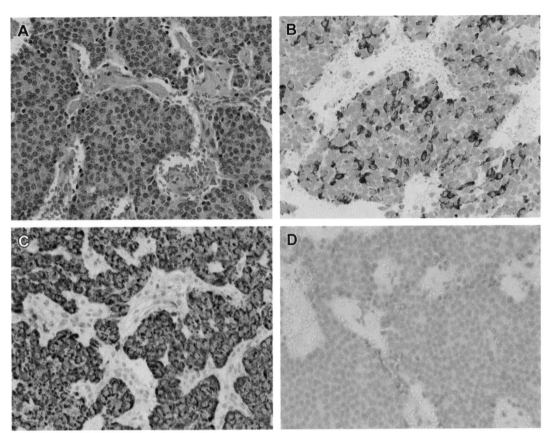

Fig. 2. IHC can help resolve differential diagnoses, which include Pan-NEN. All sections are at ×40 magnification. (*A*) Hematoxylin-eosin stain of a pancreatic neoplasm showing tumor cells growing in a solid and nestlike pattern. The tumor cells stain diffusely positive for CGA (*B*) and CAM 5.2 (*C*) and are negative for AE1/AE3 (*D*).

discussed later) and can be confused with metastatic RCC of the clear cell type (also seen in VHL).[17] Several other unusual cellular features can occasionally be seen, including black

pigmentation (usually due to melanin), spindle-type cells, rhabdoid cells, oncocytic change, and sarcomatoid change (occasionally with skeletal muscle cells). Notably, so-called naked islands of

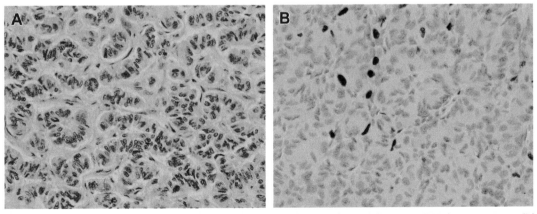

Fig. 3. Pan-NEN can show diverse architectural features. (*A*) A nonfunctioning Pan-NEN demonstrates solid, trabecular, and pseudoacinar patterns of growth within the same lesion. IHC for Ki-67 (*B*) reveals a proliferative index of 5%, grading this Pan-NEN as intermediate (grade 2). The images shown are at ×40 magnification.

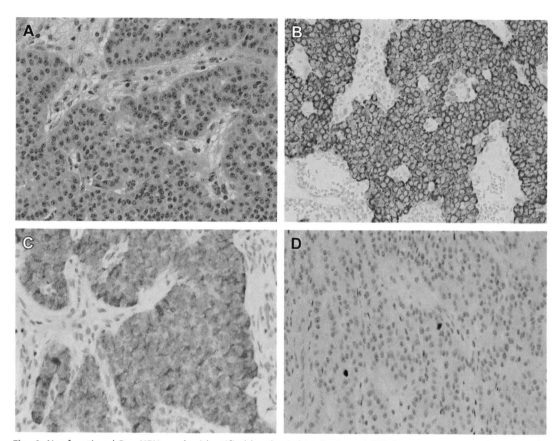

Fig. 4. Nonfunctional Pan-NEN can be identified by classic histologic and IHC features. Hematoxylin-eosin of a nonfunctional Pan-NEN (*A*). The tumor cells are diffusely positive for CGA (*B*) and synaptophysin (*C*). The Ki-67 labeling index was less than 1%, revealing this tumor to be low grade (grade 1) (*D*). (*A* and *C*), ×40; (*B* and *D*), ×20.

neoplastic cells can be found in peripancreatic adipose tissue, a feature that can be confused with invasion.

The stromal component of Pan-NEN is vascular and can be variable in both character and amount. Abundant hyaline material sometimes intervenes between nests of neoplastic cells. Calcifications can manifest as irregular masses or as psammoma bodies. Irregular calcifications of significant size can be found in both primary lesions and in metastases. Such calcifications are nonspecific, but psammoma bodies are characteristic of δ-cell tumors (somatostatinoma; discussed later). Amyloid (islet amyloid polypeptide [IAPP]) is particularly common in (although not exclusive to) β-cell, insulin-positive neoplasms. IAPP can sometimes be detected in the serum or tissues.

Most lesions have low-grade histology, with few mitoses. There are unfortunately few reliable and reproducible predictors of malignant behavior, other than the self-evident findings of distant metastases (**Fig. 6**). Relative indicators of a poor

prognosis include local invasion, gross extension into adjacent organs, vascular invasion, large size, necrosis, and increased mitotic activity. Even low-grade lesions can exhibit marked nuclear pleomorphism, and this feature does not correlate with prognosis.[15]

GRADING AND STAGING PANCREATIC NEUROENDOCRINE NEOPLASMS

GI-NENs, including Pan-NENs, generally lack reliable histologic indicators of prognosis. Evaluation of the proliferative state is becoming increasingly important in grading these lesions.[18,19] The current grading strategy endorsed by the World Health Organization, European Neuroendocrine Tumor Society, and American Joint Committee on Cancer uses either mitotic counts or IHC for Ki-67 (a pan-cell cycle marker) to stratify these lesions into a 3-grade system (**Table 1**). Currently, all GI-NENs of the tubular gut and pancreas are graded on the same system. There are some data suggesting that the behavior of Pan-NENs may differ slightly

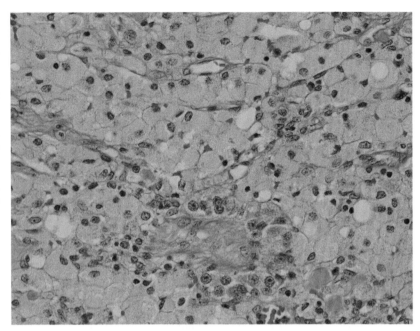

Fig. 5. Pan-NEN from a patient with VHL disease (×40 magnification). The tumor cells show clear cytoplasm, large nuclei, and conspicuous nucleoli, commonly seen in patients with VHL disease. Because patients with VHL often have RCC, distinguishing a primary Pan-NEN with clear cell change from a renal metastasis can be challenging in small biopsy specimens.

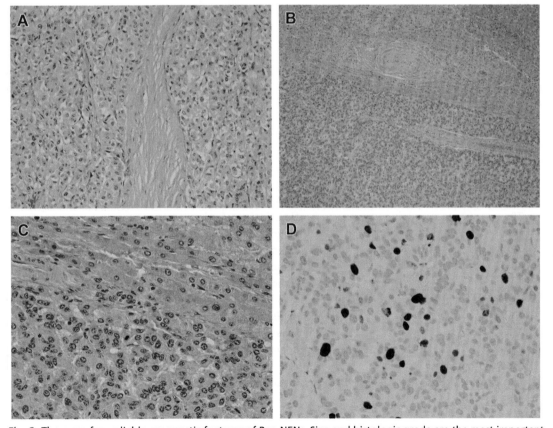

Fig. 6. There are few reliable prognostic features of Pan-NENs. Size and histologic grade are the most important prognostic markers for Pan-NEN, but metastases can occur with lesions of any grade. (*A*) Hematoxylin-eosin ×20 of a primary Pan-NEN reveals 1 mitosis per 50 high-power fields (grade 1). Metastasis of the same lesion to the liver at ×10 (*B*) and ×40 (*C*) magnifications reveals 6 mitoses per 50 high-power fields and a Ki-67 labeling index (*D*) of 10% (grade 2).

Table 1
Grading Pan-NENs

Grade	Mitoses (No. per 10 High-Power Field or 2 mm²)		Ki-67 Index (% of 2000 Cells)
G1 (low)	<2	AND	<3
G2 (intermediate)	2–20	OR	3–20
G3 (high)	>20	OR	>20

Adapted from Rindi G, Kloppel G, Alhman H, et al. TNM staging of foregut (neuro)endocrine tumors: a consensus proposal including a grading system. Virchows Arch 2006;449(4):395–401; Table 4, page 399; with permission.

from other GI-NENs, such that a Ki-67 index of less than 6% may be a more appropriate G1/G2 cutoff than less than 3%, but support for such a change is insufficient at this time to separate grading of Pan-NENs from other GI-NENs. Staging conforms to a TNM system, with the most important parameters the size of the lesion and local invasion (**Table 2**).

MOLECULAR FINDINGS AND TARGETED THERAPY

The genetics of tumor syndromes that can include Pan-NEN as a component are discussed later. Among sporadic Pan-NENs, approximately 50% exhibit aneuploidy. Ploidy itself does not correlate with malignancy, but, among malignant tumors, aneuploidy correlates with more aggressive behavior. Loss of 6q occurs more frequently in insulinoma.[20] Approximately half of sporadic Pan-NENs exhibit either loss of chromosome 11q or mutation of MEN1 (11q13).[21–23] Telomerase is absent, and DPC4/SMAD4 is rarely inactivated, in contrast to pancreatic adenocarcinoma.[24]

In addition to a role in imaging (discussed previously), SSRTs play a role in the treatment of Pan-NENs.[11,12] Octreotide or similar somatostatin analogues are administered with the goal of repressing the secretion of hormone from functional neuroendocrine cells, in particular those of gastrinoma, glucagonoma, and VIPoma. Octreotide can exacerbate symptoms due to insulinoma. As with imaging, the class of tumor (and by extension the distribution and subtype of the SSRTs) has a significant bearing on which neoplasms can be treated. There are 5 types of SSRTs (SSRT1–SSRT5), with SSRT2 (the most common type) divided into subtypes 2A and 2B.

Epidermal growth factor receptor (EGFR) expression has been correlated with tumorigenesis in several tissues. Evaluation of EGFR expression in Pan-NEN has shown varying results (25%–65%) in different studies. Among cases that do express EGFR, those with activated EGFR (P-EGFR) expression have exhibited worse prognosis than those without P-EGFR expression.[25]

Table 2
Staging of Pan-NENs

T—primary tumor	
Tx	Primary tumor cannot be assessed
T0	No evidence of primary tumor
T1	Tumor <2 cm and limited to pancreas
T2	Tumor 2–4 cm and limited to pancreas
T3	Tumor >4 cm or invading duodenum or bile duct
T4	Tumor invading adjacent organs or wall of large vessels
N—regional lymph nodes	
Nx	Regional nodes cannot be assessed
N0	No evidence of regional nodal metastasis
N1	Regional lymph node metastasis
M—distant metastasis	
Mx	Distant metastasis cannot be assessed
M0	No evidence of distant metastasis
M1	Distant metastasis

Adapted from Rindi G, Kloppel G, Alhman H, et al. TNM staging of foregut (neuro)endocrine tumors: a consensus proposal including a grading system. Virchows Arch 2006;449(4):399; with permission; and *Data from* Kloppel G, Couvelard A, Perren A, et al. ENETS Consensus Guidelines for the Standards of Care in Neuroendocrine Tumors: toward a standardized approach to the diagnosis of gastroenteropancreatic neuroendocrine tumors and their prognostic stratification. Neuroendocrinology 2009;90(2):162–6.

DIFFERENTIAL DIAGNOSIS

The differential diagnosis for Pan-NENs is usually fairly narrow and can be approached in 2 ways: conditions that mimic the clinical syndromes of functional Pan-NEN and conditions that appear histologically similar to Pan-NEN (Table 3). Functional mimics of Pan-NEN are discussed later. The most frequent histologic mimics of Pan-NEN are solid pseudopapillary carcinoma (Fig. 7A, B), acinar carcinoma (see Fig. 7C), and ductal adenocarcinoma exhibiting an unusual solid architecture. These lesions can exhibit architecture and cytology (either focally or predominantly) that appear difficult to distinguish from Pan-NEN. Other lesions, such as pancreatoblastoma or mixed endocrine-ductal carcinoma, actually contain neuroendocrine cells as a component.[8] In either scenario, increased sampling to reveal specific histologic features (eg, grooved nuclei in solid pseduopapillary neoplasms or mucin in ductal carcinoma) with or without IHC can be helpful (see Table 3). Metastatic or locally invasive NENs from outside the pancreas (small cell carcinoma, paraganglioma/extra-adrenal pheochromocytoma, and so forth) can be challenging, because they are often histologically difficult to distinguish from true Pan-NEN. IHC markers specific for the gastrointestinal (GI) tract (CDX-2) or pancreas (Isl-1) can be useful in this context.

Nesidioblastosis deserves special mention as a diagnostic challenge. Originally coined to describe the histologic appearance of neonatal pancreas in the context of hyperinsulinemic

Table 3
Differential diagnostic considerations

	Rationale	Resolution
Acinar Cell Carcinoma	Uniform cells with delicate vasculature	Butyrate esterase+, trypsin+, and PAS-D+
Solid and pseudopapillary tumors		Areas of pseudopapillae; blood lakes; grooved nuclei; CAM 5.2−, vimentin+, β-catenin+
Solid ductal adenocarcinoma	Unusual appearance can mimic Pan-NEN	Intracellular mucin, desmoplasia, CEA+, MUC1+
Paraganglioma, GI-NEN	Nonpancreatic NENs near the pancreas can look very similar to Pan-NEN	
Pheochromocytoma	Nonpancreatic NENs near the pancreas can look very similar to Pan-NEN	Abundant cytoplasm, organoid architecture, serum and urine studies
Pancreatoblastoma	Pluripotent cell lineage can exhibit neuroendocrine differentiation	Squamoid nests can be seen; CK+, trypsin+, chymotrypsin+
MEN syndromes	May include Pan-NEN	Family history and molecular genetic studies
Nesidioblastosis	Hypersecretes insulin, causing hyperinsulinemic hypoglycemia	Islets should appear normal, aside from hyperplasia and enlarged cells
Solitary fibrous tumor	Secretes IGF-2, causing hyperinsulinemic hypoglycemia (can be confused with insulinoma)	Radiology, histology
Chronic pancreatitis	Proliferating islet cells can be confused with NEN	Clinical history, gross appearance of pancreas
Mixed endocrine-ductal	Entrapped normal glands	Ductal features pertain
Metastatic small cell lung cancer (SCLC)	Can be difficult to distinguish from primary Corticotropin-secreting lesions of the pancreas	Radiology
Angiomyolipoma (PEComa)	Difficult to distinguish from liver metastases of Pan-NEN	HMB45+
Metastatic RCC	Pan-NEN with clear cell change often seen in VHL	CD10+

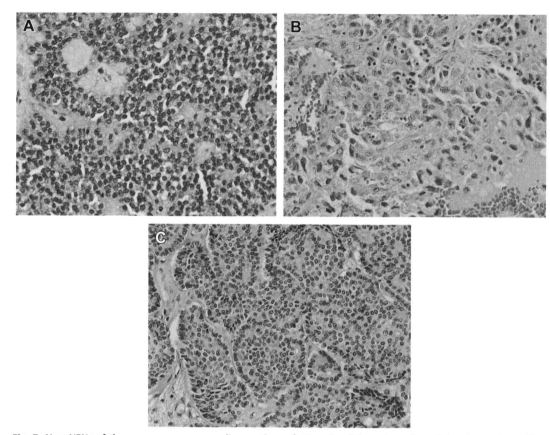

Fig. 7. Non-NENs of the pancreas can cause diagnostic confusion. A solid portion of a solid and pseudopapillary neoplasm of pancreas (*A, B*) exhibits medium-sized, relatively uniform cells and may be mistaken for Pan-NEN. The presence of myxoid connective tissue (*A*), however, is not seen in Pan-NEN. Solid and pseudopapillary neoplasm of pancreas can also show cytoplasmic eosinophilic granules (*B*), which helps distinguish these tumors from Pan-NENs. Acinar cell carcinoma (*C*) with uniformity of the cells and delicate vasculature may suggest a neuroendocrine tumor. IHC stains for chromogranin, synaptophysin, butyrate esterase, trypsin, and histochemical staining for PAS after diastase digestion helps to separate these neoplasms. All panels are shown at ×40 magnification.

hypoglycemia, the term, *nesidioblastosis*, is now more frequently applied to a reactive pancreatic islet hyperplasia and islet-cell hypertrophy, occasionally occurring after gastric bypass surgery (**Fig. 8**).[26–29] The nuclei can also become enlarged and irregular. In adults, Pan-NEN is usually a solitary lesion outside of MEN1, whereas nesidioblastosis appears multifocal. In pediatric patients, however, focal nesidioblastosis can be observed as a solitary nodule. Islets observed in nesidioblastosis should retain the same IHC properties as normal islets, including peptide hormone production.

CLINICAL CATEGORIZATION

From a clinical perspective, Pan-NEN often comes to a patient's and clinician's attention as either the cause, or one component, of a syndrome. This is a consequence of perhaps the most salient feature of Pan-NEN, which is its ability to produce functional hormone. Functional hormone production often has severe clinical consequences and associated morbidity and mortality. These clinical syndromes and their sequelae, however, also tend to bring patients to clinical attention and treatment sooner, often yielding better overall outcomes. Because each syndrome by which a patient may be afflicted can yield different diagnostic challenges and clinical outcomes, Pan-NEN is divided into categories based on the expression of functional hormone, and the type of hormone expressed, with special consideration given to lesions that may arise in the context of a genetic syndrome.

Functional Pancreatic Neuroendocrine Neoplasms

Functional Pan-NENs are recognized based on clinical syndromes resulting from functional

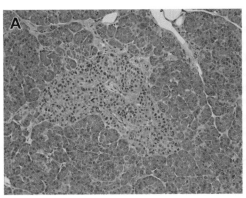 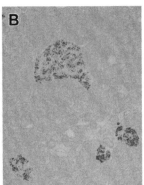 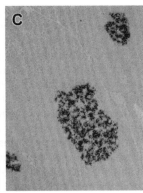

Fig. 8. Nesidioblastosis can confound a diagnosis of Pan-NEN. Patients who undergo gastric bypass surgery can develop a reactive nesidioblastosis. In a small percentage of such patients, some of the islets are markedly enlarged measuring more than 2 to 3 times the diameter of the average islet (*A*) (×20). Some islet cells have enlarged nuclei as in this image. Other findings may include islet cells budding off small pancreatic ducts and peliosis-type changes in the islets. IHC (*B*) and in situ hybridization (*C*) patterns for insulin (both at ×10 magnification) show enlargement of the islet (compare with islets within panel) but are otherwise normal, demonstrating insulin-positive cells constituting a majority of cells.

hormone produced by the neoplasm. Any of the hormones produced by normal pancreatic islet cells can be overproduced by a Pan-NEN, including insulin, glucagon, somatostatin, and pancreatic polypeptide (PP). Additionally, ectopic hormone production can also occur, including corticotropin, VIP, parathyroid-like hormone, calcitonin, and growth hormone–releasing hormone. Gastrin is unique, because it is produced by the fetal, but not the adult, pancreas. Presumably because of this property, gastrin is the most commonly secreted ectopic hormone. As with other NENs, Pan-NENs may secrete either an α or β subunit of human chorionic gonadotropin (hCG), which can be useful as a serum marker. Multiple hormones may be secreted by the same lesion. In such a scenario, multiple metastases may each secrete different functional hormones. Similarly, in cases of multiple primary lesions, each primary can potentially secrete a different hormone. IHC for hormone products can often be useful to confirm a diagnosis. If multiple hormone secretion is suspected, it is important to consider the possibility of entrapped normal islets. IHC for hormone products is nearly always nonuniform—cells vary both in their production and in their subcellular distribution of the peptides. The detection of hormonal peptide by IHC does not define the tumor as functional—the Pan-NEN is categorized as functional or nonfunctional based solely on the presence or absence of clinically detectable symptoms. Strictly speaking, nonfunctional neoplasms should be described based on their cell of origin, rather than on their presumptive hormonal product, to avoid confusion (eg, β-cell neoplasm rather than insulinoma).

β-Cell neoplasms (insulinomas)

A majority of functional Pan-NENs produce insulin. They tend to be small, solitary, and preferentially located in the head and tail of the pancreas.[30–32] Approximately 50% secrete another hormone in addition to insulin.[3] Demographically, these neoplasms slightly favor women over men and affect adults more often than children. Insulinomas are more often benign than other functional tumors or nonfunctional tumors; 90% of β-cell tumors are solitary, and of the remaining multifocal tumors, virtually all are seen in the context of MEN1; 2% of β-cell neoplasms are found outside the pancreatic parenchyma.

The Whipple triad of hyperinsulinemic hypoglycemia comprises (1) hypoglycemia (convulsions, confusion, and weakness/fatigue), (2) plasma glucose less than 3 mmol/L, and (3) symptomatic relief by glucose administration. Plasma levels of insulin, proinsulin, C-peptide, and glucose are measured and compared to demonstrate inappropriate secretion of insulin relative to plasma glucose. The syndrome is common in the context of functional insulinoma but is not universal. Furthermore, although functional β-cell tumor is the most common cause of the hyperinsulinemic hypoglycemia, other lesions can cause a similar clinical picture: solitary fibrous tumors (either benign or malignant) secrete IGF-2, causing a hyperinsulinemic effect, and nesidioblastosis can hypersecrete insulin.[26]

Histologically, β-cell neoplasms most commonly exhibit a solid or gyriform architecture, usually without glands (see **Fig. 2**). Amyloid (IAPP) is a characteristic, fairly specific finding, but is unfortunately not common. IHC for insulin usually positive, although it generally does not stain as strongly as in non-neoplastic islets. IHC for proinsulin is positive in approximately half of cases. Insulin and proinsulin can both sometimes be detected in serum. β-Cell tumors often show defects in the production and secretion of functional hormone, which can result in lesions that stain positively for insulin or proinsulin by IHC, despite lacking clinical symptoms of hyperinsulinemia. Again, it is important to reserve the term insulinoma for lesions that induce hyperinsulinemic symptoms. Staining for chromogranin A (CGA) is generally weaker than in other Pan-NENs.

The prognosis of β-cell lesions is good—10% or less become malignant, with older male patients carrying the greatest risk. As with other forms of Pan-NEN, size greater than 2 cm, local invasion, angioinvasion, increased mitoses, and greater than 2% Ki-67 index are all poor prognostic signs. Nesidioblastosis, in addition to being a potential source of hyperinsulinemic hypoglycemia, can also serve as the focus of origin of Pan-NEN.[26]

β-Cell neoplasms (insulinomas)

- Whipple triad of hyperinsulinemic hypoglycemia

- Majority of functional Pan-NENs

- Small, solitary, and usually in head or tail of pancreas

- Approximately 50% secrete other hormones in addition to insulin

- Most tumors benign

- Amyloid (IAPP) is a specific finding

- Prognosis usually excellent after surgical excision

G-cell neoplasms (gastrinomas)

Gastrinoma (Zollinger-Ellison) syndrome manifests with hypersecretion of gastric acid leading to ulcers (usually multiple) of the gastric, duodenal, and/or jejunal mucosa. Approximately one-third of patients may present with chronic diarrhea. Although sporadic G-cell tumors are more likely to form within the pancreas (hence, their classification within the Pan-NENs), multifocal G-cell tumors in the context of MEN more frequently develop within the duodenum (and occasionally the stomach).[33] Occasionally, intra-abdominal tumors in other locations (possibly representing metastasis from an occult primary) can produce hypergastrinemia. Fasting serum gastrin, both at baseline and after stimulation by subcutaneous injection of secretin, can be used to diagnose gastrinoma.

Gastrinomas represent a significant proportion (20%) of functional Pan-NENs. Multifocality is more common than in other Pan-NEN subtypes, especially as a part of MEN1, a context in which as much as 25% of gastrinomas arise. In MEN1, most gastrinomas arise in the duodenum rather than the pancreas. Sporadic gastrinomas are almost always solitary and malignant. G-cell Pan-NENs have a high risk of malignancy at any size, with pancreatic G-cell NENs carrying a worse prognosis than those in the duodenum. Usually, G-cell Pan-NEN exhibits a solid and/or glandular histologic architecture, and the cells appear more like gastrin-producing cells (eg, of the stomach) than pancreatic islet cells. IHC is usually positive for gastrin, but in situ hybridization can occasionally confirm a nonfunctional G-cell Pan-NEN. Non-neoplastic islets within the pancreas can show reactive nesidioblastosis.

G-cell neoplasms (gastrinomas)

- Associated with hypersecretion of gastric acid (Zollinger-Ellison syndrome)

- Approximately one-third of patients present with chronic diarrhea

- Develops most frequently in duodenum

- Multiple tumors common, especially with MEN1

- Most sporadic tumors are malignant

α-Cell tumors (glucagonoma)

α-Cell tumors (see **Fig. 1**) are usually solitary and large at the time of presentation (mean of 7 cm). They most frequently arise within the pancreatic tail and often present with degenerative changes.[34] IHC is usually weak or negative for glucagon. PP is often coexpressed in α-cell tumors. α-Cell tumors have a greater tendency toward malignant transformation than other Pan-NENs, with up to 70% of patients having metastases at the time of presentation. The clinical glucagonoma syndrome (hypersecretion of glucagon from Pan-NEN) mainly affects adult women. It can manifest clinically with any combination of severe weight loss, necrolytic migratory erythema (a skin rash predominantly below the waist), angular stomatitis, sore red tongue, deep vein thrombosis, abnormal glucose tolerance test, normocytic normochromic anemia, depression, and tendency to develop overwhelming infection. Nonfunctional α-cell tumors are more often small, multifocal, and benign.

Necrolytic migratory erythema deserves special mention, because it may be examined microscopically. It manifests in up to 70% of patients with glucagonoma, as a direct consequence of hyperglucagonemia. The syndrome is not specific to glucagonoma, however, also occurring in the context of pancreatitis, celiac disease, and cirrhosis. The rash begins as erythema, progressing to superficial blisters, which spread outward with central clearing. The rash heals in 1 to 2 weeks, resolving with hyperpigmentation but without true scarring. Histologically, the rash is characterized by epidermal necrolysis, liquefaction necrosis of the granular cell layer, and subcorneal clefting or blister formation.

α-Cell neoplasms (glucagonomas)

Solitary and large, usually in pancreatic tail, with greater tendency for malignancy

IHC weak or negative for glucagon

Hypersecretion syndrome can include necrolytic migratory erythema, angular stomatitis, sore red tongue, and deep vein thrombosis

---

δ-Cell tumors (somatostatinomas)
The somatistatinoma syndrome is more rare, more clinically subtle, and less well defined than most of the other functional Pan-NEN syndromes. It can include diabetes, indigestion, steatorrhea, cholecystolithiasis, indigestion, hypochlorhydria, and occasionally anemia. The inhibitory nature of somatostatin yields the more subtle and variable clinical findings. The tumors are usually solitary and malignant.[35] There is a female predilection, and 65% of patients have metastases on presentation. δ-Cell tumors are most often found in the head of the pancreas but can be found elsewhere, including the duodenal wall. Psammoma bodies are common, particularly in duodenal lesions. Synaptophysin is a more reliable IHC marker than chromogranin in these lesions, but staining for both markers should be performed in the workup of any Pan-NEN.

δ-Cell neoplasms (somatostatinomas)

Usually solitary and malignant

Somatostatin syndrome rare and subtle

Psammoma bodies are a specific finding

Synaptophysin more reliable than chromogranin

Pancreatic polypeptide secreting tumors
Pan-NENs secreting PP alone are rare, but PP is commonly secreted by multihormone-producing neoplasms. Symptoms associated with hypersecretion of PP alone are nonspecific, including weight loss, diarrhea, abdominal pain or cramping, and GI bleeding. Hyperplasia and hypersecretion of non-neoplastic PP cells can also be seen in the setting of Pan-NENs of any subtype.

Vasointestinal peptidoma
VIP is not normally produced by pancreatic islets, and, as with other functional Pan-NENs secreting ectopic hormones, VIPomas are rare. Despite their low frequency, they comprise up to 80% of diarrheogenic Pan-NENs. Thus, watery diarrhea in the absence of infectious causes or gastric hypersecretion should prompt consideration of VIPoma. Hypersecretion of VIP often causes electrolyte disturbances and dehydration, although the osmolar gap is usually normal. VIPomas are virtually indistinguishable histologically from gastrinoma, except (perhaps self-evidently) by IHC for VIP versus gastrin. These tumors often secrete more than one hormone product, including PP (discussed previously), calcitonin, and α-hCG. In children, VIP hypersecretion often occurs in ganglioneuroma rather than Pan-NEN.[36]

Serotoninoma (carcinoid tumors)
The serotonin-secreting Pan-NENs are similar to GI-NENs seen in the tubular GI system, including the capacity to produce the carcinoid or serotonin syndrome, usually caused by metastasis to the liver. The syndrome consists of flushing, diarrhea, and bronchoconstriction. Serotoninomas exhibit strong argentaffinity, in contrast to all other Pan-NENs, which are argyrophilic. Serotoninomas tend to be large at the time of detection.[37]

Ectopic hormone production
In addition to the normal suite of pancreatic hormones, functional Pan-NENs may also secrete hormones not normally found in pancreatic islets, including growth hormone (GH), GH-releasing hormone (GHRH), corticotropin-releasing hormone, hCG, calcitonin, antidiuretic hormone, melanocyte-stimulating hormone, neurotensin, secretoneurin, parathyroid hormone–like polypeptide, secretogranin II, inhibin, activin, prohormone convertases 2 and 3, and metallothionein. Acromegaly can be a dramatic clinical presentation for a hormone secreting tumor, but greater than 98% of cases are due to pituitary neoplasms, and half of the remainder are due to neuroendocrine tumors of the lung. Consideration of a GH- or GHRH-secreting Pan-NEN (or GI-NEN) should be considered after negative radiologic evaluation of other sites. So-called

small cell tumors of the pancreas sometimes secrete corticotropin (like their counterparts in the lung) and may resemble primitive neuroectodermal tumor (PNET) histologically. Distinguishing these lesions from lung metastases is challenging histologically, and a suspected diagnosis of primary pancreatic small cell carcinoma should prompt thorough clinical and radiologic evaluation for a lung primary.[38]

Nonfunctioning Neoplasms

Nonfunctioning Pan-NEN is misleading, because these tumors may produce hormone (detectable in serum or by IHC), and the hormone may be functional. Because the excess hormone does not cause symptoms in these patients, however, the lesions are described as nonfunctional. Immunohistochemically, these neoplasms are often positive for multiple hormones.[39]

Malignant potential of nonfunctional lesions closely correlates with the size at the time of presentation. Lesions less than 2 cm are generally nonmalignant, with lesions less than 0.5 cm classified as benign microadenomas. Although lesions 2 cm or greater are more likely malignant, they are still generally low-grade neoplasms with few mitoses (see Fig. 4).

These lesions occur most often in the head of the pancreas. Nonfunctional Pan-NENs can show a variety of cytologic and architectural features, which should not be surprising because the specific cell types from which they originate are diverse. Nonfunctional α-cell tumors are often small and multiple, with a gyriform architecture. Glucagon is often strongly immunoreactive, despite the nonfunctional nature of the lesion. Nonfunctional α-cell tumors are nearly always benign.

Familial Pancreatic Neuroendocrine Neoplasms—Multiple Endocrine Neoplasia, Type 1; von Hippel-Lindau Disease; Neurofibromatosis 1; Tuberous Sclerosis

Presentation of multiple primary Pan-NEN lesions or Pan-NEN in the context of other extrapancreatic neoplasms should always prompt the consideration of a genetic tumor syndrome. Multiple Pan-NENs are almost always seen in the context of one of the multiple endocrine neoplasia (MEN) subtypes.

Multiple endocrine neoplasia type 1 (Werner syndrome)
MEN1 is due to mutations in the *MEN1* gene (11q13).[22] The syndrome includes Pan-NEN as well as adenomas of the anterior pituitary, and chief cell hyperplasia of the parathyroid glands. The pancreatic neoplasms are most frequently G-cell tumors (50% of cases), followed by β-cell

tumors (30%), VIP cell tumors (12%), and α-cell tumors (<5%). The clinical syndrome includes symptoms from lesions in all 3 anatomic locations, so, in addition to symptoms from the specific Pan-NEN, patients may experience primary hyperparathyroidism and acromegaly or hypopituitarism. Less commonly, NENs of the tubular GI tract, lungs, and thymus (carcinoids), as well as adenomas or nodular hyperplasia of the adrenal cortex and thyroid, can be seen. Other lesions may include multiple soft tissue lipomas, multiple leiomyomas at various sites, and Ménétrier disease of the stomach. In contrast to sporadic Pan-NEN, Pan-NEN in the context of MEN1 presents at a younger age, is often multifocal, and is more likely cystic (Fig. 9). Although not a diagnostic feature of other MEN syndromes, Pan-NEN is known to occur in such a background.

von Hippel-Lindau
VHL is inherited in an autosomal-dominant manner on chromosome 3. The syndrome includes tumors in multiple organ systems, including RCC, vascular tumors in the central nervous system, pheochromocytoma, endolymphatic sac tumors in the ear, and cystadenoma in the epididymis. The pancreas is most often affected by cysts and serous cystadenomas that can cause symptoms but do not have malignant potential. Pan-NEN does also occur in an estimated 17% of patients and presents some unique challenges in the context of VHL. In addition to the possibility of cystic lesions in the pancreas potentially confounding the diagnosis, Pan-NENs in VHL often shows clear cell change. Because RCC is also common in VHL, there can be difficulty distinguishing Pan-NEN from a clear-cell RCC metastasis. Pan-NEN in VHL is almost always nonfunctional, tends to be multiple, and often presents alongside pheochromocytoma in the same patient.

Neurofibromatosis 1
Neurofibromatosis 1 (NF1) is caused by a defect in the neurofibromin gene and is inherited in an autosomal-dominant manner on chromosome 17q11.2.[22] Approximately 1% of patients afflicted with NF1 exhibit Pan-NEN as part of their syndrome. In the context of NF1, the Pan-NEN is usually a functional or nonfunctional δ-cell neoplasm (somatostatinoma), often involving the duodenum, although other subtypes have been identified as well.

Tuberous sclerosis complex
Tuberous sclerosis complex (TSC) is an autosomal dominant condition caused by a germline mutation in the TSC1 or TSC2 gene.[22] Clinically, it manifests with the formation of multiple tumors—predominantly hamartomas and benign tumors but also

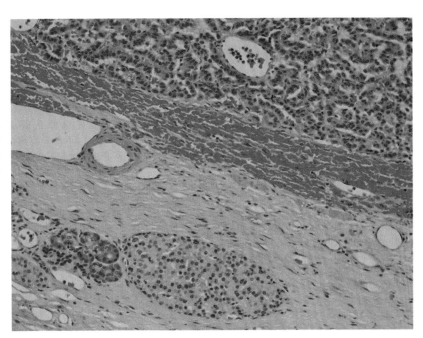

Fig. 9. Pan-NEN from a nonfunctioning tumor, shown at ×40 magnification. In addition to the large tumor in the upper half of the field, the small nest of islet-like cells in the lower portion of the field is most likely a microscopic focus of islet cell tumor, as recent studies have demonstrated in patients with MEN1.

malignancies—in multiple organs. Commonly affected organs include the skin, kidney, and lungs. Pan-NEN is not a pathognomonic finding nor even common in TSC patients, with an incidence of approximately 2%. Still, it is approximately 10,000 times more common in TSC patients than in the general population. Additionally, the widely held assumption that pancreatic neoplasms in the context of TSC are angiomyolipomas seems false. Suspected pancreatic lesions in the appropriate clinical context warrant evaluation for Pan-NEN. Pan-NEN in the context of TSC, like MEN1, is often cystic and presents at a younger age than sporadic Pan-NEN. Presentation with a solitary lesion, however, is much more common in TSC than it is in MEN1.

TREATMENT AND PROGNOSIS

Medical management of Pan-NEN focuses on symptomatic relief and is dependent on the clinical syndrome and biological properties of the individual lesion or lesions.[11,12] It is often most important in the presurgical management of syndromic effects. The clinical syndromes due to glucagonoma, gastrinoma, and VIPoma can all be successfully treated by somatostatin analogues (octreotide or lantreotide). In contrast, these drugs may either ameliorate or exacerbate the symptoms of insulinoma. Diazoxide and thiazide drugs are often used in medical management of hyper-insulinemia.

Monitoring of disease progression in functional Pan-NENs includes serial assessment of serum hormone levels. Serum levels of CGA can also be monitored for disease progression but can be elevated in the context of renal or hepatic disease as well. CGA is not particularly sensitive for the purposes of early disease detection. Other serum markers that have been proposed or seen limited clinical use include neuron-specific enolase, PP, α- or β-hCG, and pancreastatin (a degradation product of CGA).

The gold standard treatment of an isolated Pan-NEN is surgical resection. Lesions often present after they have invaded locally or metastasized, in particular nonfunctional Pan-NEN or neoplasms that produce vague symptoms, such as somatostatinoma. Delayed detection, increased invasion, and the anatomy of the pancreas and surrounding structures can thus make resection difficult, if not completely infeasible. For these reasons, resectability rates have been maximally estimated at 65%. Pancreaticoduodenectomy and distal or subtotal pancreatectomy are the most common surgical options. Recently, more effort has been made to undertake laparoscopic and pancreas-sparing procedures (enucleation and midpancreas resection), when possible. Isolated insulinoma, the most common manifestation of Pan-NEN, is usually curable by enucleation or partial pancreatectomy. In the case of suspected insulinoma without a preoperatively identifiable lesion, intraoperative US may be warranted.

The slow-growing nature of most Pan-NENs necessitates long-term follow-up, even in the context of an apparently successful surgery. Pan-NEN in context of multiple tumor syndromes is more complex, because the tumors tend to recur, and Pan-NEN may only be one of several therapeutic concerns for the patient.

Metastatic disease, depending on the clinical context, may be treated by tumor debulking, partial hepatic resection, hepatic embolization, radiofrequency ablation, chemotherapy, medical therapy, or some combination thereof. Pan-NENs can be slow growing, so debulking may significantly improve symptoms, despite the presence of metastatic disease. Isolated liver metastases also tend to grow slowly and can selectively resected or ablated in the appropriate context.

Octreotide can be useful in managing symptoms of functional metastases and may also have a tumoristatic effect. Interferon is also often administered for tumoristatic properties. Radiolabeled octreotide analogues are under investigation as targeted radiotherapy, based on the same biological properties that permit SSRT scintigraphy. Unlike NENs of the tubular GI tract, Pan-NEN has been shown to be responsive to traditional chemotherapeutic regimens, including streptozocin, 5-fluorouracil, and doxorubicin, usually in combination. Angiogenesis inhibitors and mTor inhibitors are among the novel chemotherapeutic approaches that have shown some promise in clinical trials and may be used (particularly in combination therapy) increasingly in the future.

SUMMARY

Despite the low incidence of Pan-NENs, the biological potential to secrete functional hormone lends them a special clinical importance. Small lesions, even grossly and radiologically undetectable ones, can present with severe syndromes. Although not all Pan-NENs are functional, even nonfunctional lesions may be detected or treated by making use of their unique biological properties. Nonfunctional Pan-NENs may pose diagnostic challenges to practicing pathologists, including between other malignancies (solid and pseudopapillary or acinar cell carcinoma) and nonmalignant conditions (chronic pancreatitis or nesidioblastosis). Clinical, histologic, IHC, and genetic findings can help resolve the differential and lead to appropriate management and better clinical outcomes.

REFERENCES

1. Rosai J. Pancreas and ampullary region. In: Rosai J, editor. Rosai and Ackerman's surgical pathology, vol. 1, 10th edition. Edinburgh (United Kingdom); New York: Mosby; 2011. p. 1005–55.

2. Thompson LD, Heffess CS. Pancreas. In: Sternberg SS, Mills SE, Carter D, editors. Sternberg's diagnostic surgical pathology, vol. 2. Philadelphia: Wolters Kluwer Health/Lippincott Williams & Wilkins; 2010. p. 1431–91.

3. Heitz P, Komminoth P, Perren A, et al. Pancreatic endocrine tumours: introduction. In: DeLellis RA, Lloyd R, Heitz P, et al, editors. Pathology and genetics: tumours of endocrine organs. World Health Organization classification of tumours, vol. 8. Lyon (France): IARC Press; 2004. p. 177–82.

4. van Eeden S, Offerhaus GJ. Historical, current and future perspectives on gastrointestinal and pancreatic endocrine tumors. Virchows Arch 2006;448(1): 1–6.

5. Verbeke CS. Endocrine tumours of the pancreas. Histopathology 2010;56(6):669–82.

6. Oberg K, Eriksson B. Endocrine tumours of the pancreas. Best Pract Res Clin Gastroenterol 2005; 19(5):753–81.

7. Pereira PL, Wiskirchen J. Morphological and functional investigations of neuroendocrine tumors of the pancreas. Eur Radiol 2003;13(9):2133–46.

8. Raman SP, Hruban RH, Cameron JL, et al. Pancreatic imaging mimics: part 2, pancreatic neuroendocrine tumors and their mimics. AJR Am J Roentgenol 2012;199(2):309–18.

9. Lewis RB, Lattin GE Jr, Paal E. Pancreatic endocrine tumors: radiologic-clinicopathologic correlation. Radiographics 2010;30(6):1445–64.

10. Tan EH, Tan CH. Imaging of gastroenteropancreatic neuroendocrine tumors. World J Clin Oncol 2011; 2(1):28–43.

11. Kulke MH, Bendell J, Kvols L, et al. Evolving diagnostic and treatment strategies for pancreatic neuroendocrine tumors. J Hematol Oncol 2011;4:29.

12. Metz DC, Jensen RT. Gastrointestinal neuroendocrine tumors: pancreatic endocrine tumors. Gastroenterology 2008;135(5):1469–92.

13. Ligneau B, Lombard-Bohas C, Partensky C, et al. Cystic endocrine tumors of the pancreas: clinical, radiologic, and histopathologic features in 13 cases. Am J Surg Pathol 2001;25(6):752–60.

14. Goh BK, Ooi LL, Tan YM, et al. Clinico-pathological features of cystic pancreatic endocrine neoplasms and a comparison with their solid counterparts. Eur J Surg Oncol 2006;32(5):553–6.

15. Zee SY, Hochwald SN, Conlon KC, et al. Pleomorphic pancreatic endocrine neoplasms: a variant commonly confused with adenocarcinoma. Am J Surg Pathol 2005;29(9):1194–200.

16. Singh R, Basturk O, Klimstra DS, et al. Lipid-rich variant of pancreatic endocrine neoplasms. Am J Surg Pathol 2006;30(2):194–200.

17. Hoang MP, Hruban RH, Albores-Saavedra J. Clear cell endocrine pancreatic tumor mimicking renal cell carcinoma: a distinctive neoplasm of von

Hippel-Lindau disease. Am J Surg Pathol 2001; 25(5):602–9.

18. Klimstra DS, Modlin IR, Coppola D, et al. The pathologic classification of neuroendocrine tumors: a review of nomenclature, grading, and staging systems. Pancreas 2010;39(6):707–12.

19. Rindi G, Kloppel G, Alhman H, et al. TNM staging of foregut (neuro)endocrine tumors: a consensus proposal including a grading system. Virchows Arch 2006;449(4):395–401.

20. Speel EJ, Richter J, Moch H, et al. Genetic differences in endocrine pancreatic tumor subtypes detected by comparative genomic hybridization. Am J Pathol 1999;155(6):1787–94.

21. Larson AM, Hedgire SS, Deshpande V, et al. Pancreatic neuroendocrine tumors in patients with tuberous sclerosis complex. Clin Genet 2012;82(6):558–63.

22. Lodish MB, Stratakis CA. Endocrine tumours in neurofibromatosis type 1, tuberous sclerosis and related syndromes. Best Pract Res Clin Endocrinol Metab 2010;24(3):439–49.

23. Callender GG, Rich TA, Perrier ND. Multiple endocrine neoplasia syndromes. Surg Clin North Am 2008;88(4):863–95, viii.

24. Perren A, Saremaslani P, Schmid S, et al. DPC4/Smad4: no mutations, rare allelic imbalances, and retained protein expression in pancreatic endocrine tumors. Diagn Mol Pathol 2003;12(4):181–6.

25. Papouchado B, Erickson LA, Rohlinger AL, et al. Epidermal growth factor receptor and activated epidermal growth factor receptor expression in gastrointestinal carcinoids and pancreatic endocrine carcinomas. Mod Pathol 2005;18(10):1329–35.

26. Anlauf M, Wieben D, Perren A, et al. Persistent hyperinsulinemic hypoglycemia in 15 adults with diffuse nesidioblastosis: diagnostic criteria, incidence, and characterization of beta-cell changes. Am J Surg Pathol 2005;29(4):524–33.

27. Raffel A, Krausch MM, Anlauf M, et al. Diffuse nesidioblastosis as a cause of hyperinsulinemic hypoglycemia in adults: a diagnostic and therapeutic challenge. Surgery 2007;141(2):179–84 [discussion 185–6].

28. Tsujino M, Sugiyama T, Nishida K, et al. Noninsulinoma pancreatogenous hypoglycemia syndrome: a rare case of adult-onset nesidioblastosis. Intern Med 2005;44(8):843–7.

29. Meissner T, Wendel U, Burgard P, et al. Long-term follow-up of 114 patients with congenital hyperinsulinism. Eur J Endocrinol 2003;149(1):43–51.

30. Chen X, Cai WY, Yang WP, et al. Pancreatic insulinomas: diagnosis and surgical treatment of 74 patients. Hepatobiliary Pancreat Dis Int 2002;1(3):458–61.

31. Grant CS. Insulinoma. Best Pract Res Clin Gastroenterol 2005;19(5):783–98.

32. Komminoth P, Perren A, Oberg K, et al. Insulinoma. In: DeLellis RA, Lloyd R, Heitz P, et al, editors. Pathology and genetics: tumours of endocrine organs. World Health Organization classification of tumours, vol. 8. Lyon (France): IARC Press; 2004. p. 183–6.

33. Komminoth P, Perren A, Oberg K. Gastrinoma. In: DeLellis RA, Lloyd R, Heitz P, et al, editors. Pathology and genetics: tumours of endocrine organs. World Health Organization classification of tumours, vol. 8. Lyon (France): IARC Press; 2004. p. 191–4.

34. Kloppel G, Komminoth P, Perren A, et al. Glucagonoma. In: DeLellis RA, Lloyd R, Heitz P, et al, editors. Pathology and genetics: tumours of endocrine organs. World Health Organization classification of tumours, vol. 8. Lyon (France): IARC Press; 2004. p. 187–8.

35. Dayal Y, Oberg K, Perren A, et al. Somatostatinoma. In: DeLellis RA, Lloyd R, Heitz P, et al, editors. Pathology and genetics: tumours of endocrine organs. World Health Organization classification of tumours, vol. 8. Lyon (France): IARC Press; 2004. p. 189–90.

36. Peng SY, Li JT, Liu YB, et al. Diagnosis and treatment of VIPoma in China: (case report and 31 cases review) diagnosis and treatment of VIPoma. Pancreas 2004;28(1):93–7.

37. Osamura RY, Oberg K, Speel EJ, et al. Serotonin-secreting tumour. In: DeLellis RA, Lloyd R, Heitz P, et al, editors. Pathology and genetics: tumours of endocrine organs. World Health Organization classification of tumours, vol. 8. Lyon (France): IARC Press; 2004. p. 198.

38. Osamura RY, Oberg K, Perren A. ACTH and other ectopic hormone producing tumours. In: DeLellis RA, Lloyd R, Heitz P, et al, editors. Pathology and genetics: tumours of endocrine organs. World Health Organization classification of tumours, vol. 8. Lyon (France): IARC Press; 2004. p. 199–200.

39. Klimstra DS, Perren A, Oberg K. Non-functioning tumours and microadenomas. In: DeLellis RA, Lloyd R, Heitz P, et al, editors. Pathology and genetics: tumours of endocrine organs. World Health Organization classification of tumours, vol. 8. Lyon (France): IARC Press; 2004. p. 201–4.

40. van Eeden S, de Leng WW, Offerhaus GJ, et al. Ductuloinsular tumors of the pancreas: endocrine tumors with entrapped nonneoplastic ductules. Am J Surg Pathol 2004;28(6):813–20.

Familial Endocrine Syndromes

Peter M. Sadow, MD, PhD[a,b], Nicole M. Hartford, CT(ASCP)[a], Vania Nosé, MD, PhD[a,b],*

KEYWORDS

- Endocrine tumors • Familial endocrine syndrome • Inherited neoplasm syndrome
- Inherited tumor syndrome • Multiple endocrine neoplasia • Familial diseases

ABSTRACT

Endocrine tumors may present as sporadic events or as part of familial endocrine syndromes. Familial endocrine syndromes (or inherited tumor/neoplasm syndromes) are characterized by multiple tumors in multiple organs. Some morphologic findings in endocrine tumor histopathology may prompt the possibility of familial endocrine syndromes, and these recognized histologic features may lead to further molecular genetic evaluation of the patient and family members. Subsequent evaluation for these syndromes in asymptomatic patients and family members may then be performed by genetic screening.

genetic evaluation of the patient and family members. Subsequent evaluation for these syndromes in asymptomatic patients and family members may then be performed by genetic screening.

OVERVIEW

Endocrine tumors may present as sporadic events or as part of familial endocrine syndromes.[1] The first description of a multiple endocrine neoplasia (MEN) syndrome was in early 1900s. Aided largely by the discovery of causative genes and advanced molecular diagnostics, familial endocrine syndromes, largely emerging over the past century, are becoming more clearly elucidated.[2] Familial endocrine syndromes (or inherited tumor/ neoplasm syndromes) are characterized by multiple tumors in multiple organs. In addition to the classic syndromes, such as MEN syndromes (Box 1), newer described entities have been identified, such as hyperparathyroidism–jaw tumor (HPT-JT) syndrome and pheochromocytoma-paraganglioma syndromes, among others. Some morphologic findings in endocrine tumor histopathology may prompt the possibility of familial endocrine syndromes, and these recognized histologic features may lead to further molecular

PITUITARY

Pituitary adenomas are benign neoplasms with excessive proliferation of any subtype of pituitary cells. Clinically, these tumors can give rise to profound disease due to hormonal aberration or to visual disturbance due to mass effect. Pituitary adenomas are predominantly monoclonal and various studies show that the tumor development is related to defects in oncogenes and tumor suppressor genes. These tumors can be present as an isolated event or as part of a familial endocrine syndrome.[3]

PITUITARY ADENOMA AS PART OF FAMILIAL ENDOCRINE SYNDROMES

Currently, approximately 5% of all pituitary adenoma cases have a family history of pituitary adenomas (Table 1), mainly because of MEN type 1 (MEN1) and Carney complex (CNC).[4–6] Familial isolated pituitary adenoma (FIPA) was described in 1999.[7]

Multiple Endocrine Neoplasia Type 1

The first pituitary adenoma in MEN1 was originally described in 1903 by Erdheim[2] at the autopsy of a patient concurrently exhibiting a pituitary adenoma and 3 enlarged parathyroid glands. Over the past century, knowledge of MEN1 in both its molecular genetic underpinnings and its clinical implications was important for the clinical management of MEN patients.

[a] Pathology Service, Massachusetts General Hospital, Boston, MA, USA; [b] Department of Pathology, Harvard Medical School, Boston, MA, USA
* Corresponding author. Pathology Service, Massachusetts General Hospital, Boston, MA, USA.
E-mail address: vnose@partners.org

Surgical Pathology 7 (2014) 577–598
http://dx.doi.org/10.1016/j.path.2014.08.008
1875-9181/14/$ – see front matter © 2014 Elsevier Inc. All rights reserved.

Box 1
Classic multiple endocrine neoplasia syndromes

MEN1 gene; 11q13:

  PHPT (>90%): occurs at younger age than sporadic counterpart

  Pituitary tumors (10%–60%): mean age of diagnosis is 38

  1. PRLs: 60%

  2. GH-secreting adenomas: 10%

  3. Others

  Enteropancreatic tumors (60%–70%)

  1. Familial Zollinger-Ellison syndrome, with gastrin-producing tumors, multiple duodenal tumors

  2. Insulinomas

  3. Glucagonomas, VIPomas

  4. Nonfunctioning

  Gastric enterochromaffin-like proliferations: multiple lesions

  Thymic or bronchial endocrine tumors (5%–10%)

  Adrenal cortical tumors (20%–40%)

  1. Aldosterone-producing tumors

  2. Cortisol-producing tumors

  Soft tissue tumors

  Central nervous system tumors

MEN2A (*RET* gene; 10q11.2): 70%–80% of cases of MEN2 precursor lesions

  Neoplastic CCH and adrenal medullary hyperplasia

  MTC (90%–l00%)

  Pheochromocytoma (10%–60%)

  Parathyroid hyperplasia or adenoma (10%–30%)

MEN2B (*RET* gene; 10q11.2): ∼5% of cases of MEN2 precursor lesions

  Neoplastic CCH and adrenal medullary hyperplasia

  MTC (100%): aggressive form associated with CCH

  Pheochromocytoma (40%–60%)

  Mucosal neuromas of lips, tongue, eyelids (>70%)

  Ganglioneuromatosis of the intestine (>60%)

  Marfanoid habitus (100%)

  Medullated corneal nerve fibers (>60%)

CNC (*PRKAR1A* gene; 17q22-24):

  PPNAD (>25%) with Cushing syndrome

  Mucocutaneous pigmented lesion (100%)

  Myxomas (40%–90%)

  Multiple thyroid follicular adenomas (75%)

  Pituitary GH-producing adenoma (10%)

  Large cell calcifying Sertoli cell tumor

  Psammomatous melanotic schwannoma

  Osteochondromyxoma

Table 1
Pituitary adenomas as part of familial endocrine syndromes

Syndrome	Gene/Chromosome Location	Pituitary Pathology
MEN1	*MEN1*/11q13	Prolactin or GH-producing adenoma, nonfunctional adenoma
McCune-Albright	*GNAS1*/20q13.3	GH-producing adenoma, GH-prolactin hyperplasia
FIPA	*AIP*/11q13.3	GH-producing adenoma, prolactin-producing adenoma
CNC	*PRKAR1A*/17q22-24	GH-producing adenoma
MEN4	CDKN1B/12p13.1-p12	GH-producing adenoma
Isolated familial somatotropinoma	*AIP*/11q13.3	GH-producing adenoma

MEN1 is an autosomal dominant disease characterized by multifocal endocrine tumors affecting the anterior pituitary gland, parathyroid, endocrine pancreas, adrenal cortices, and endocrine-based lesions of other organs (see **Box 1**). MEN1 has an age-related penetrance and variable expression. The *MEN1* gene is localized on chromosome 11q13. It consists of 10 exons, which encode the 610 amino acid protein, menin. Menin is a cell cycle–dependent intranuclear protein thought to facilitate cell growth and differentiation during embryogenesis and postnatal life.[8-10] Homozygous inactivation of the *MEN1* gene is lethal early during embryogenesis.

Pituitary adenomas are integral components of the MEN1 syndrome.[2,11] The prevalence of pituitary adenomas in MEN1 has varied from 20% to 60% depending on the study. Mean age of onset of pituitary adenomas is 38 ± 15 years, with rare occurrences in children younger than 5 years.

Pituitary adenomas in MEN1 are usually hormonally active,[12] with prolactinomas (PRLs) most commonly seen (60%), followed by growth hormone (GH)-secreting (10%), corticotropin-secreting (5%), and nonsecreting (15%) lesions (see **Box 1**). Non–mass-related symptoms are hormone related, and female patients with PRLs often present with amenorrhea, infertility, and galactorrhea, whereas male patients often present with hypogonadism.

The pathology findings of pituitary adenoma in MEN1 are not different from those seen in sporadic pituitary adenomas. A majority of MEN1 patients exhibit a single adenoma and multicentricity seems extremely rare.[1,13] Although there is no convincing evidence for the isolated diffuse hyperplasia of onecell type, PRL or GH cell hyperplasia of the peritumoral parenchyma has been described.[14]

Treatment of pituitary adenoma in MEN1 is identical to that applied in sporadic counterparts. The clinical outcome is also similar to the sporadic counterparts.[15]

Carney Complex

CNC is characterized by mucocutaneous pigmented lesions, myxomas, endocrine tumors, and pigmented schwannomas within other tumors (see **Box 1**).[16,17] CNC is inherited as an autosomal dominant trait. Mutations of the *PRKARIA* gene on chromosome 17 were identified.[18] Another chromosome 2 (2p15-p16) locus was identified in CNC.[19] Several endocrine glands can be involved simultaneously, including pituitary, adrenal, and thyroid (see **Box 1**). Acromegaly occurs in only 10% of CNC cases, but approximately 75% of patients have elevation in GH or prolactin levels. Lesions in the pituitary gland range from pituicyte hyperplasia to multiple microadenomas to invasive macroadenoma. Microscopically, CNC-related acromegaly is distinguished by multifocal hyperplasia of somatomammotropic cells within nonadenomatous pituitary tissue. CNC should be considered for patients who present with acromegaly and typical multifocal hyperplasia of pituitary tissue. The treatment of individual manifestations of CNC does not differ from sporadic cases.

Familial Isolated Pituitary Adenomas

FIPA is an autosomal dominant disease characterized by early onset and often aggressive pituitary tumor growth.[20] In 15% of FIPA families, germline mutation and loss of heterozygosity have been described in the *aryl hydrocarbon receptor interacting protein (AIP)* gene.[21] Patients with *AIP* mutations have an overwhelming predominance of PRL (41%) and somatotropinoma (30%) (see **Table 1**) with early presentation.[22] Patients with *AIP* mutations have a poorer response to therapy.

Other Syndromes Associated with Pituitary Adenomas: McCune-Albright Syndrome, Isolated Familial Somatotropinoma Syndrome, MEN4

> **Key points**
>
> - In summary, pituitary adenomas in inherited tumor syndromes may differ from their sporadic counterparts not only in genetic basis but also in clinical and pathologic characteristics (see Table 1).[1]
> - Thus, early recognition of these inherited syndromes is important.

PARATHYROID

Primary hyperparathyroidism (PHPT) refers to an increase of serum calcium and parathyroid hormone concentrations. It is one of the most common endocrine diseases. Clinically, the symptoms of PHPT are well known as "moans, groans, stones, and bones." PHPT may result from genetically heterogeneous diseases, including hyperplasia, adenoma, or rarely, carcinoma. Approximately 95% of cases occur as sporadic disorders. PHPT occurring at younger age, however, clinically should raise the suspicion of a familial syndrome.

PRIMARY HYPERPARATHYROIDISM AS PART OF INHERITED TUMOR SYNDROMES

The familial form of hyperparathyroidism (Table 2) is found in many autosomal dominant disorders, including MEN1, and MEN2, hereditary HPT-JT syndrome, familial isolated hyperparathyroidism (FIHP), neonatal severe hyperparathyroidism,

familial hypocalciuric hypercalcemia (FHH), autosomal dominant mild hyperparathyroidism, and familial hypercalcemia and hypercalciuria.[1,13,23] With clinical and genetic surveillance, however, patients with familial hyperparathyroidism are often identified earlier. The diagnosis is made based on elevated parathyroid hormone and elevated serum calcium levels.

Multiple Endocrine Neoplasia Type 1

PHPT is the main MEN1-associated endocrinopathy. It occurs in 90% of individuals between ages 20 and 25 years. Although MEN1-associated PHPT is frequently asymptomatic for a long period of time, patients often manifest with hypercalcemia, and the prevalence of disease approaches 100% by 40 years of age.

The histologic findings are the same as those described for hyperplasia occurring in a nonfamilial setting. Grossly, all 4 glands are generally enlarged and the cut surface is tan, soft, and homogenous. Microscopically, the glands are hypercellular with a paucity of intraparenchymal fat. The predominant cell type is the chief cell, which has faintly eosinophilic cytoplasm and a centrally placed round monotonous nucleus. In patients with known MEN1, a diagnosis of parathyroid adenoma should not be used, because all glands are likely to be affected, and recurrent disease is common in patients with MEN1 after partial parathyroidectomy. MEN1 patients should be treated with surgery, either total multiple parathyroidectomy with autotransplantation or subtotal resection of 3.5 parathyroid glands.[24]

Multiple Endocrine Neoplasia Type 2A

MEN type 2 (MEN2) is an autosomal dominant inherited tumor syndrome caused by *RET* gene mutations.[25] It is characterized by the presence of endocrine tumors variably involving the

Table 2
Hyperparathyroidism as part of familial endocrine syndromes

Syndrome	Gene/Chromosomal Location	Parathyroid Pathology
MEN1	*MEN1*/11q13	Parathyroid hyperplasia and/or adenoma
MEN2A	*RET*/10q11.2	Multiglandular hyperplasia
HPT-JT	*HRPT2*/1q25-q32	Cystic parathyroid adenomas and carcinomas
FHH	*CaSR*/3q13.3-q21	Mild parathyroid hyperplasia
Familial hypercalcemia and hypercalciuria	*CaSR*/3q13.3-q21	Parathyroid hyperplasia and/or adenoma
FIHP	*CaSR*/3q13.3-21 *HRPT2*/1q25-q32	Multiglandular hyperplasia, parathyroid carcinoma
Neonatal severe PHPT	*CaSR*/3q13.3-21	Primary hyperplasia

thyroid, parathyroid, and adrenal glands (see Box 1). Abnormalities involving nonendocrine organs may be present. The *RET* gene encodes a tyrosine kinase receptor.[26] Specific codon mutations in *RET* correlate with disease phenotypic and severity.[27]

PHPT is part of MEN2A, whereas it is rare in MEN2B. The prevalence of parathyroid disease in MEN2A is approximately 20% to 30%. Occasionally, it is the first clinical presentation of MEN2A. The pathologic findings include single or multiple parathyroid gland hyperplasias. Parathyroid hyperplasia in the patient with *RET* mutation should be treated with surgery. Genetic testing of *RET* mutations and clinical surveillance allows earlier intervention in patients with medullary thyroid carcinoma (MTC) or pheochromocytomas.

Hereditary Hyperparathyroidism–Jaw Tumor

HPT-JT syndrome is a rare, autosomal dominant familial disorder linked to the chromosomal region of 1q25-q32 (*HRPT2* locus).[28] It is characterized by familial hyperparathyroidism, ossifying jaw fibromas, and renal neoplastic and non-neoplastic abnormalities. Hyperparathyroidism is present in all patients, at a median age of 36.3 years.[29] Pathologically, parathyroid enlargement for these tumors is primarily due to multiple adenomas, some of which are cystic; 10% to 15% of these patients develop parathyroid carcinoma. The HPT-JT syndrome has frequent single-gland parathyroid involvement and an increased risk of carcinoma. Thus, early diagnosis of HPT-JT is important, and genetic testing is essential.[30]

Familial Isolated Hyperparathyroidism

FIHP is a rare cause of parathyroid tumors lacking other endocrine anomalies.[31] FIHP is an autosomal dominant disorder, which may represent an early stage of either the MEN1 or HPT-JT.[32,33] Mutations of *MEN1* and *HRPT2* genes have been identified. Screening for other tumors associated with MEN1 and HPT-JT should be performed for the diagnosis of FIHP. These patients present with profound hypercalcemia more frequently compared with MEN1. Loss of parafibromin expression is a distinguishing marker of parathyroid involvement in FIHP. Limited parathyroidectomy is an effective treatment because single-gland involvement often occurs.

Neonatal Severe Hyperparathyroidism

Neonatal severe hyperparathyroidism is a disorder characterized by hypercalcemia as a result of diffuse chief cell hyperplasia.[34] It occurs only rarely in childhood under the age of 6 months and is characterized by multigland parathyroid hyperplasia rather than adenoma. It is caused by homozygous inactivating mutations of the *calcium-sensing receptor gene* (*CaSR*). Total parathyroidectomy in the neonatal period is necessary for survival of the patient.

Familial Hypocalciuric Hypercalcemia

FHH is inherited as an autosomal dominant trait with mild to moderate hypercalcemia accompanied by few symptoms. This is the most common cause of hereditary hypercalcemia. FHH prevails in approximately half of the cases of hypercalcemia during the first 2 decades of life. Heterozygous loss of function mutations cause FHH in which the lifelong mild hypercalcemia is generally asymptomatic.[35] Histologically, the parathyroid glands removed from FHH patients are normal or occasionally hyperplastic.[36]

Key points

- In summary, although only approximately 5% of cases presenting with hyperparathyroidism are familial, its recognition in the setting of autosomal dominant inherited tumor syndromes is important.

- Identification is especially important in MEN1, MEN2A, and HPT-JT.

- Clinical surveillance and genetic testing are necessary screens for prevention/detection of malignancy or fatal complications of familial endocrine syndromes.

THYROID

Thyroid cancer accounts for approximately 2% of all malignant tumors. The incidence of thyroid cancer has increased, however, at a rate higher than most other cancers.[1,13,37] Thyroid carcinomas may derive from follicular cell origin (95%) or calcitonin-producing C cells (5%).[38] Approximately 5% of patients with thyroid tumors with follicular cell origin have familial disease, which increases to 25% in patients with MTCs.[39,40]

Familial syndromes are classified as familial non-MTC (FNMTC) and familial MTC (FMTC).[1,13,41]

FOLLICULAR CELL NEOPLASM AS PART OF AN INHERITED TUMOR SYNDROME

FNMTC is further subclassified into 2 subgroups (**Box 2**): familial syndromes characterized by a predominance of nonthyroidal tumors and familial tumor syndromes characterized by a predominance of non-MTC (NMTC).[1,41–43]

Familial Syndromes Characterized by a Predominance of Nonthyroidal Tumors

The first group of FNMTCs includes familial syndromes characterized by a predominance of nonthyroidal tumors, such as PTEN hamartoma tumor syndrome (PHTS)/Cowden syndrome (CS), familial adenomatous polyposis (FAP), CNC type 1, Pendred syndrome, and Werner syndrome (**Table 3**).

PTEN hamartoma tumor syndrome

PHTS is a group of syndromes characterized by germline inactivating mutations of the *PTEN* tumor suppressor gene, which is located on chromosome 10q22-23. PHTS includes CS, Bannayan-Riley-Ruvalcaba syndrome (BRRS), Proteus syndrome, and Proteus-like syndrome.[44] Affected individuals develop both benign and malignant tumors in a variety of tissues, including thyroid, in two-thirds of PHTS patients. Breast carcinoma and thyroid carcinoma are the 2 most common malignancies present in individuals with CS.

Thyroid pathologic findings in patients with PHTS that normally affect the follicular cells include multinodular goiter, multiple adenomatous nodules (MANs), follicular adenoma (**Fig. 1**), follicular thyroid carcinoma, and, less frequently, papillary thyroid carcinoma (PTC).[1,13,45] Follicular carcinoma is an important feature in CS and BRRS. According to the diagnostic criteria for CS, follicular carcinoma is a major criterion, and multinodular goiter, adenomatous nodules, and follicular adenomas are minor criteria, with a frequency of 50% to 67%.

MANs are characteristic findings in these syndromes and present grossly as multiple, firm, yellow-tan, well-circumscribed nodules.[46] These nodules are multicentric, bilateral, well-circumscribed, unencapsulated features similar to follicular adenomas. The authors' believe, from

Table 3
Follicular cell neoplasm as part of familial endocrine syndromes

Disorder	Gene/Chromosomal Location	Thyroid Pathology
FAP	*APC*/5q21	PTC CMV
PHTS	*PTEN*/10q23.31	MANs Follicular adenoma Follicular carcinoma PTC Lymphocytic thyroiditis CCH
CNC	*PRKAR1A*/17q23-q24	MANs Follicular carcinoma Follicular adenoma PTC
Pendred syndrome	*PDS*/7q31	Multinodular goiter
Werner syndrome	*WRN*/8p12	PTC Anaplastic thyroid carcinoma

Fig. 1. PHTS: histopathology of a nodule from a patient with Cowden syndrome (CS) shows an encapsulated follicular adenoma. These adenomas are usually present in a background of MANs and lymphocytic thyroiditis (hematoxylin & eosin [H&E], magnification ×200).

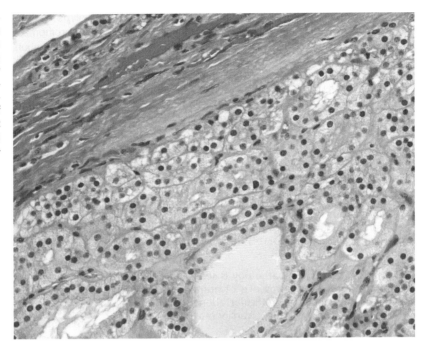

experience, that the morphologic findings of MAN should be considered a possible major criterion in CS and BRRS.[46] These tumors are more frequently multicentric. A majority of carcinomas arise in a background of MAN.[1,13,47] Although cancer risk in BRRS was expected to be similar to the general population, the authors found 4 cases of follicular thyroid carcinoma (67%), showing that this type of carcinoma was more frequent in the pediatric population, and believe that these patients should follow the same management guidelines as for CS.[1,13] Immunohistochemistry for PTEN shows loss of staining of the follicular cells (**Fig. 2**).

Fig. 2. PHTS: immunohistochemistry for PTEN in a thyroidectomy specimen in a patient with CS shows loss of staining of the follicular cells (PTEN immunostain, magnification ×200).

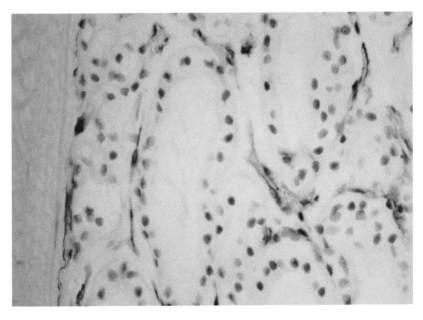

MTC is not considered part of the spectrum of PHTS; however, earlier studies[1,13] have identified C-cell hyperplasia (CCH) in individuals affected with this syndrome.[45,46,48,49] Most studies have failed to show a consistent genotype-phenotype relationship in PHTS. Careful phenotyping gives further support for the suggestion that BRRS and CS are actually one condition, presenting at different stages.

Key points

- In summary, the presence of numerous adenomatous nodules, in a background of lymphocytic thyroiditis, should raise suspicion for a diagnosis of PHTS in younger patients.

- Multinodular thyroid pathology is seen and characterized by the presence of numerous adenomatous nodules, follicular adenomas, and follicular thyroid carcinomas in PHTS.[1,13,46]

Familial adenomatous polyposis
FAP is an inherited autosomal dominant syndrome caused by germline mutations in the *adenomatous polyposis coli (APC)* gene, characterized by clinically innumerable adenomatous colonic polyps.[50] Although the development of colorectal carcinoma stands out as the most prevalent complication, FAP is a multisystemic disorder. Extracolonic manifestations of FAP include upper gastrointestinal tract polyps, osteomas, epidermal cysts, desmoid tumors, hamartomas, hepatoblastomas, congenital hypertrophy of the retinal pigmented epithelium, and thyroid tumors.[1,13,51] PTC occurs in approximately 12% of patients. Adolescents and young women with FAP are at particular risk for developing thyroid carcinomas, and their chances of being affected are approximately 160 times higher than that of normal individuals (PTC occurs with a frequency of approximately 10 times than expected for sporadic PTC).[52]

Thyroid carcinomas associated with FAP are usually bilateral and multifocal, with histologic features different from sporadic tumors. The cribriform-morular variant (CMV) of PTC (**Figs. 3** and **4**) was first described as an FAP-associated thyroid carcinoma.[1,13,53] Inactivation of the *APC* tumor suppressor gene initiates colorectal neoplasia and is also involved in FAP-related thyroid tumors. Mutations of the *APC* gene lead to a truncated protein that lacks the β-catenin binding site and, therefore, cannot degrade β-catenin. One of the biochemical activities associated with the APC protein is down-regulation of transcriptional activation mediated by β-catenin (**Fig. 5**).

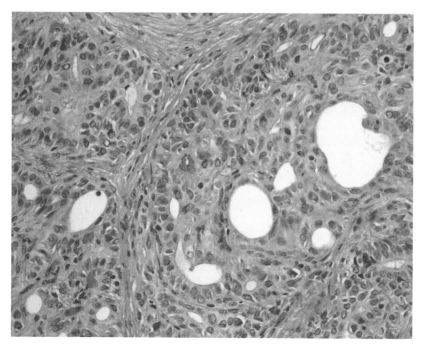

Fig. 3. CMV-PTC: photomicrograph of a thyroid tumor from a patient with FAP shows a cribriform patterned tumor with focal solid component and areas of fibrosis (H&E, magnification ×200).

Fig. 4. CMV-PTC: photomicrograph of a thyroid tumor from a patient with FAP demonstrates the characteristic peculiar nuclear clearing within the squamoid morules (H&E, magnification ×400).

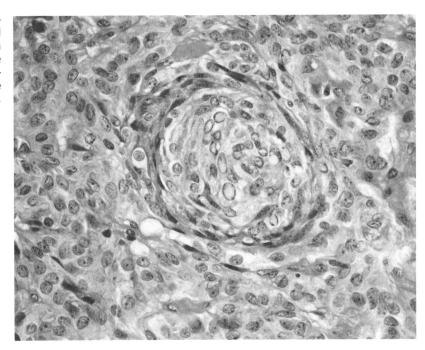

Key points

- The distinct CMV-PTC seen in FAP-related thyroid carcinomas is unusual in sporadic PTC.

- Any patient with a pathologic diagnosis of CMV-PTC should be evaluated for FAP and mutation of the *APC* gene.

Carney complex

CNC is an autosomal dominant disease characterized by diversely pigmented skin and mucosal lesions as well as a variety of endocrine neoplasms (pituitary adenoma, pigmented nodular adrenal disease, Sertoli-Leydig cell tumors, and thyroid tumors) (see **Box 1**). Patients with CNC may share similar components with other familial MEN. The

Fig. 5. CMV-PTC: immunohistochemistry for β-catenin in a thyroid tumor from a patient with FAP shows nuclear and cytoplasmic staining within the morular and cribriform components of the tumor (beta catenin immunostein, magnification ×400).

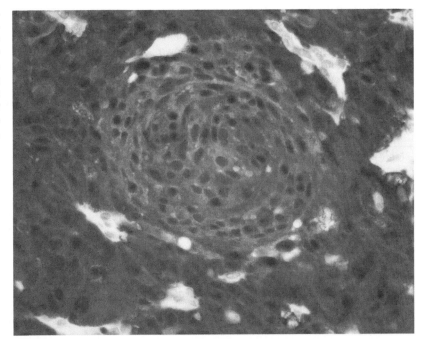

thyroid is usually multinodular, with MANs, follicular adenomas, and carcinoma in up to 15% of patients.[38,54]

Pendred syndrome

Pendred syndrome, also known as deaf-mutism and goiter, is the most common hereditary syndrome associated with bilateral deafness as a result of mutation in PDS gene on chromosome 7q21.[55] The PDS gene encodes the protein pendrin, which is a sodium-independent chloride/iodine transporter. Pendrin is involved in iodine transport at apical cell membrane of thyrocytes.[56] Mutation of this gene results in impairment of organification of iodide and, clinically, patients present with thyroid nodular hyperplasia and possible hypothyroidism.

Werner syndrome

Werner syndrome, an autosomal recessive disease, is caused by mutations in WRN gene on chromosome 8p11-12. WRN encodes a protein involved in DNA repair and replication. Clinically, Werner syndrome is associated with both an elderly appearance of skin as well as various malignancies, including well-differentiated thyroid carcinoma.[57]

Familial Tumor Syndromes Characterized by a Predominance of Nonmedullary Thyroid Carcinoma

The second group of NMTCs includes familial syndromes characterized by a predominance of NMTCs: pure familial (f) PTC with or without oxyphilia; fPTC with papillary renal cell carcinoma; and fPTC with multinodular goiter (Table 4).[1,13] FNMTC is diagnosed when 3 or more family members have NMTC in the absence of other known associated syndromes. Statistical estimates suggest that a grouping of 2 family members with NMTC could represent the concurrence of sporadic tumors but thyroid tumors in 3 or more members in kindred, or a diagnosis of PTC in men and children, is more suggestive of a familial predisposition.[58,59] FNMTC is now recognized as a distinct clinical entity and accounts for approximately 10% of all follicular cell origin thyroid carcinomas. FNMTC has a high incidence of multifocality and association with multiple benign nodules. FNMTC patients have shorter disease-free survival than do sporadic disease patients because of frequent locoregional recurrence.[60,61] The genetic inheritance of FNMTC remains unknown, but it seems to be an autosomal dominant mode.

1. fPTC is characterized by multicentric tumors and MAN with or without oxyphilia. fPTC enriched in thyroid carcinoma with oxyphilia has been mapped to chromosomal region 19p13, and FNMTC without oxyphilia has been mapped to chromosomal region 19p13.31. Tumor-specific loss of heterozygosity is found in sporadic follicular thyroid carcinoma with and without oxyphilia at both chromosome regions 19p13 and 2q21.32.
2. The FNMTC type 1 syndrome (mapped to chromosomal region 2q21) is characterized by PTC without any distinguishing pathologic features and without an obvious increase in frequency of nonthyroidal neoplasm in kindred members.[62]
3. fPTC associated with renal papillary neoplasia presents with the usual classic variant of PTC and with no special features.[63] The papillary renal neoplasia syndrome (fPTC/PRN), mapped to chromosomal region 1q21, includes not only PTC and the expected benign thyroid nodules but also PRN and possibly other malignancies.
4. In familial multinodular goiter syndrome, which is mapped to chromosome region 14q, some patients may develop an associated PTC.[64]

Key point

- PTCs in these syndromes are usually classic variant, without any specific morphologic characteristics.

Table 4
Familial endocrine syndromes characterized by a nonmedullary thyroid carcinoma

Disorder	Gene/Chromosomal Location	Thyroid Pathology
fPTC with oxyphilia	(TCO) Unknown/19p13.2	PTC with or without oxyphilia, multicentric
fPTC without oxyphilia	Unknown/19p13.2	Classic PTC
fPTC with papillary renal cell neoplasia	Unknown/1q21	Classic PTC
fPTC	Unknown/2q21	Classic PTC
Familial multinodular goiter with PTC	Unknown/14q	PTC in a background multinodular cyst formation

Medullary Thyroid Carcinoma as Part of Familial Endocrine Syndromes

MTC arises from the calcitonin-producing C cells of the thyroid and represents approximately 5% of all thyroid carcinomas.[65] MTCs occur in sporadic or hereditary (25% of cases) forms (MEN2 syndromes) (Table 5). Pathologically, the MTCs in MEN2 are usually preceded by CCH (Figs. 6 and 7), and these tumors are usually bilateral and multicentric. The distinguishing clinical and pathologic findings of sporadic and FMTCs are summarized in Table 6.

MEN2 is a group of syndromes resulting from *RET* mutation, including MEN2A, MEN2B, and familial thyroid medullary carcinoma. MEN2A is associated with pheochromocytoma and parathyroid hyperplasia, whereas MEN2B is associated with marfanoid habitus, mucosal neuromas, ganglioneuromatosis, pheochromocytoma, and rarely parathyroid disease (see Box 1).

The *RET* gene is a 21-exon gene that encodes a tyrosine kinase receptor. MEN2 is caused by germline autosomal dominant gain-of-function mutations in the *RET* gene. Mutations resulting in strong kinase activity are associated with more aggressive MTC. The American Thyroid Association (ATA) has recently developed a risk stratification based on the genotype.[66] Level D mutations were found to carry the highest risk for aggressive MTC, and level A mutations were found to carry the least risk for aggressiveness. The ATA also developed an age recommendation for prophylactic thyroidectomy depending on *RET* mutation (Table 7).

Multiple endocrine neoplasia type 2A

MEN type 2A (MEN2A) is an autosomal dominant syndrome associated with MTC, pheochromocytoma, and hyperparathyroidism. Clinically, although MTC is rarely observed in patients younger than 10 years, the disease prevalence starts to increase with age. By 13 years of age, disease prevalence is approximately 25% and continues to increase to approximately 70% at 70 years. The possibility of developing MTC is almost 100% with this syndrome (see Box 1). Mutations causing MEN2A in most cases often affect the cysteine-rich extracellular domain. The most common mutation is in codon 634 of exon 11 (ATA level C).

Multiple endocrine neoplasia type 2B

MEN type 2B (MEN2B) is characterized by MTC, pheochromocytoma, ganglioneuromatosis, and marfanoid body habitus, among other features (see Box 1).[1,13] Hyperparathyroidism is rare. Clinically, MEN2B is associated with aggressive forms of MTC. It occurs early in life, before 5 to 10 years of age. The disease is often associated with positive lymph nodes and distant metastases at diagnosis.

Mutations in codon 918 of exon 16 have been identified in approximately 95% of patients with MEN2B. On rare occasions, mutations in codon 883 of exon 15 are associated with MEN2B as well. These 2 mutations are associated with the youngest age of onset, highest risk of metastasis, and increased mortality (ATA level D).

Familial medullary thyroid carcinoma

Risk for MTC may be inherited independently from its association with other endocrine syndromes/tumors. Clinically, the diseases often occur at a later age with a more favorable prognosis. The mutations often affect codons 609, 611, 618, and 620 of exon 10 (ATA level A).

The ATA has made recommendations for prophylactic thyroidectomy depending on the codon of *RET* mutation (see Table 7).

Table 5
Familial medullary thyroid carcinoma

	MEN2B	MEN2A	Familial Medullary Thyroid Carcinoma
Age at diagnosis of MTC	Infancy to <5 y	<35 y	~50 y
Incidence	Most develop medullary carcinoma	>90% Develop medullary carcinoma	100% Develop medullary carcinoma
Presentation	Aggressive form; preventable by prophylactic thyroidectomy	Up to 70% have already lymph nodes metastases at time of diagnosis	Medullary carcinoma is the only neoplasm
% of MEN2 syndromes	~5	~70–80	~10–20

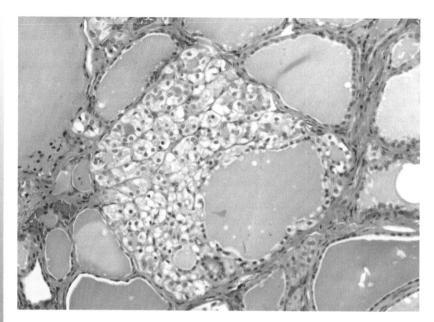

Fig. 6. CCH in a patient with MEN2A: photomicrography illustrates the CCH readily identified on hematoxylin-eosin–stained slides, usually seen in cases of neoplastic CCH (H&E, magnification ×100).

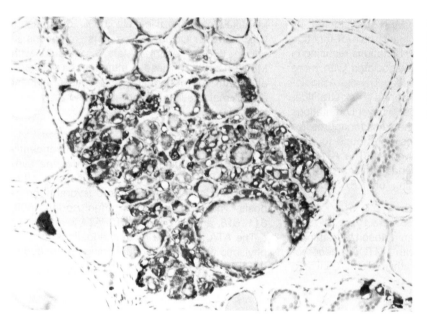

Fig. 7. CCH in a patient with MEN2A: immunohistochemistry for calcitonin highlights the CCH in a diffuse and nodular pattern (calcitonin immunostain, magnification ×100).

Table 6
Features distinguishing sporadic from familial medullary thyroid carcinoma

	Sporadic	Familial
Laterality	Unilateral	Bilateral
Tumors	Solitary	Multicentric
Associated with CCH	No/unknown	Yes
Neoplastic CCH	Rare	Frequent (~100%)
Lymph nodes metastases at time of diagnosis	Usually present	May be present

Key points

- In summary, MTC in the setting of familial endocrine syndromes often presents at a younger age; pathologically, tumors are often bilateral and multicentric with associated CCH.

- *RET* mutations should be identified in family members.

- Carriers of this high risk of mutation are candidates for prophylactic thyroidectomy and close follow-up.

ADRENAL CORTEX

Adrenal cortical tumors affect 1% to 4% of the population and up to 10% in autopsy materials. They can be non-neoplastic (such as cortical nodules, primary pigmented nodular adrenocortical disease [PPNAD], and macronodular adrenocortical hyperplasia) or neoplastic (adenoma and carcinoma). Hormonally active lesions may result in symptoms of hypercortisolism or hyperaldosteronism or lesions may be hormonally inactive (incidentalomas). Most neoplastic tumors are benign adenomas. Although adrenocortical carcinomas are rare, with estimated prevalence between 4 to 12 per million in adults, prognosis of adrenocortical carcinoma has traditionally been poor, with a 5-year survival rate below 30%.[67]

ADRENOCORTICAL TUMOR AS PART OF FAMILIAL ENDOCRINE SYNDROMES

The cause of adrenocortical tumorigenesis is poorly understood, but there are some well-defined susceptibilities for heritable malignancy in some familial syndromes.[68] Study of genetic syndromes associated with adrenocortical tumors, such as Beckwith-Wiedemann, Li-Fraumeni, McCune-Albright, CNC, and MEN1 (**Table 8**), has shed light on the molecular basis of tumorigenesis.[69]

Adrenocortical Tumor in Beckwith-Wiedemann Syndrome

Beckwith-Wiedemann syndrome is characterized by congenital malformation, overgrowth, and tumor predisposition. It is the most common overgrowth syndrome. Patients often present with exomphalos, macroglossia, and gigantism.[70] Adrenal gland pathology includes cytomegaly of the adrenal fetal cortex and adrenal cortical carcinoma. The molecular alterations on chromosome

Table 8
Adrenocortical tumor as part of familial endocrine syndrome

Syndrome	Gene/Chromosomal Location	Adrenal Pathology
Beckwith-Wiedemann	*CDKN1C*/11p15.5	NH, ACA, ACC
Li-Fraumeni	*TP53*/17p13.1	ACC
MEN1	*MEN1*/11q13	ACA, ACC
McCune Albright	*GNAS1*/20q13.3	NH, ACA
CNC	*PRKAR1A*/17q23-q24	ACA, PPNAD
NF1	*NF1*/17q11.2	ACC
FAP	*APC*/5q21	ACA, ACC
Lynch or hereditary nonpolyposis colorectal cancer	Mismatch repair proteins genes (*MSH2, MSH6, MLH1, PMS2*)/ Multiple	ACC (at least 5% of ACC are associated with lynch syndrome)
Congenital adrenal hyperplasia	*CYP21*/6p21.3	NH, ACA, ACC

Abbreviations: ACA, adrenal cortical adenoma; ACC, adrenal cortical carcinoma; NH, nodular hyperplasia.

11p15.5 have been identified in 80% of patients. Early diagnosis of this syndrome is important because of the increased risk of malignancy, including hepatoblastoma, neuroblastoma, and adrenocortical carcinoma.

Adrenocortical Tumor in Li-Fraumeni Syndrome

Li-Fraumeni syndrome is a rare autosomal dominant syndrome linked with germline *TP53* mutations. It is associated with a high risk of malignancies, including sarcoma, brain tumors, and premenopausal breast carcinoma. Adrenocortical carcinoma is the main pathology finding in the adrenal gland in this syndrome (**Figs. 8** and **9**). The median age of onset of adrenocortical carcinoma is 3 years.[71]

Primary Pigmented Nodular Adrenocortical Disease in Carney Complex

CNC is a familial multiple neoplasia and lentiginosis syndrome. The specific adrenal pathology is PPNAD (a primary bilateral adrenal disorder leading to Cushing syndrome). PPNAD is characterized, clinically, by a corticotropin-independent bilateral adrenocortical hyperfunction without obvious neoplastic changes. The nodules are multiple, small, and pigmented with internodular cortical atrophy (**Fig. 10**). Microscopically, the tumor consists of large cortical cells with abundant cytoplasmic lipofuscin pigment (**Fig. 11**). Genes linked with this syndrome are on chromosome 17 (*PRKARIA* gene) and chromosome 2.

PARAGANGLIA AND ADRENAL MEDULLA

The adrenal medulla and the paraganglia originate from the neural crest and are neuroendocrine organs and tissues. They secrete catecholamine and peptides in response to sympathetic or parasympathetic neural stimulation. The main tumors arising from these organs are paragangliomas. Pheochromocytomas are reserved for intra-adrenal tumors only. Paragangliomas occur at all ages, with 90% occurrence in adults and 10% occurrence in children.[1]

PHEOCHROMOCYTOMAS AND EXTRA-ADRENAL PARAGANGLIOMAS AS PART OF FAMILIAL ENDOCRINE SYNDROMES

Approximately 70% of tumors are sporadic and up to 30% of paragangliomas arise in a setting of inherited tumor syndromes with underlying genetic mutations (**Table 9**).[1,72] In contrast to sporadic tumors, the pheochromocytomas in the setting of familial endocrine syndromes are often multiple and bilateral. In some of the familial syndromes, pheochromocytomas may coexist with extra-adrenal paragangliomas. Thus, the findings of more than one paraganglioma indicate appropriate genetic testing and family history.

Adrenal Medullary Hyperplasia and Pheochromocytoma in Multiple Endocrine Neoplasia Type 2

MEN2 is characterized by the development of bilateral and multicentric adrenal medullary

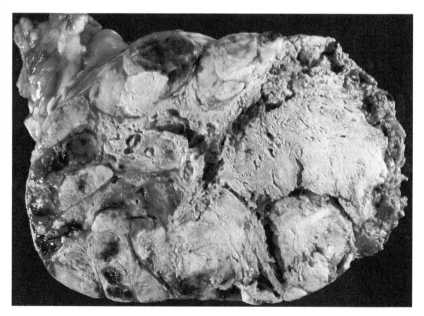

Fig. 8. Adrenal cortical carcinoma: this gross photograph shows a bulky, irregularly shaped tumor with extensive areas of necrosis, degenerative changes, and hemorrhage. The tumors are associated with specific familial syndromes, such as Beckwith-Wiedemann, Li-Fraumeni, MEN1, CNC, and Lynch syndromes.

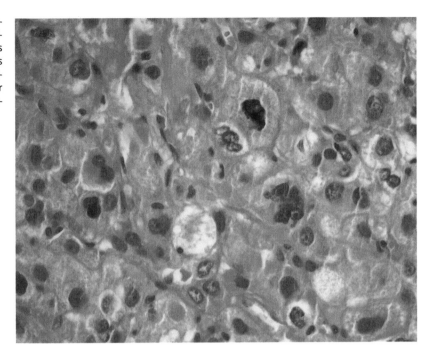

Fig. 9. Adrenal cortical carcinoma in a patient with Li-Fraumeni syndrome shows large pleomorphic cells and numerous mitotic figures, including a tripolar mitosis (H&E, magnification ×600).

hyperplasia and pheochromocytoma in addition to hyperparathyroidism and MTC (discussed previously). Extra-adrenal paragangliomas are rare, however, in these syndromes. Germline *RET* mutations are causative genes in MEN2A, 2B, and FMTCs. MEN2-related pheochromocytoma has distinct eosinophilic globules (**Fig. 12**).

Paragangliomas in Neurofibromatosis Type 1 and von Hippel–Lindau Disease

Pheochromocytomas occur in 0.1 % to 5.7% of patients with neurofibromatosis type 1 (NF1) and 10% to 30% of those with von Hippel–Lindau (VHL) disease. Germline *NF1* and *VHL* gene mutations are identified in those syndromes. Pathologically, there is no evidence that pheochromocytomas are different from sporadic ones (**Fig. 13**).

Pheochromocytoma and Paragangliomas in Familial Paraganglioma Syndromes

Familial paraganglioma syndromes (hereditary paraganglioma-pheochromocytoma syndromes) are characterized by multiple pheochromocytomas and paragangliomas in an autosomal

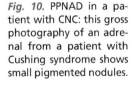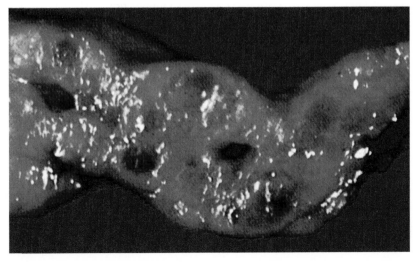

Fig. 10. PPNAD in a patient with CNC: this gross photography of an adrenal from a patient with Cushing syndrome shows small pigmented nodules.

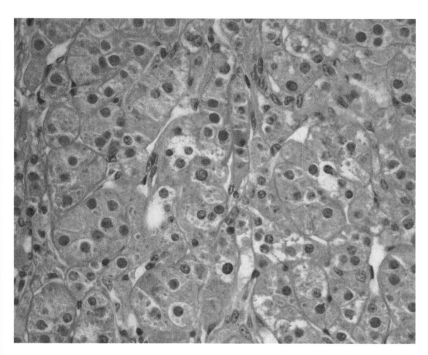

Fig. 11. PPNAD: the intranodular cells have lipid-depleted eosinophilic cytoplasm and with finely granular lipofuscin pigment and with focal accumulation of pigment (H&E, magnification ×400).

dominant manner. Extra-adrenal parasympathetic paragangliomas are located predominantly in the head and neck and most of them are nonsecretory. Sympathetic paragangliomas are often located in the thorax, abdomen, and pelvis and are often secretory. Symptoms result either from catecholamine hypersecretion or mass effect. Diagnosis of familial paraganglioma

Table 9
Pheochromocytomas and paragangliomas as part of familial endocrine syndromes

Syndrome	Gene	Tumors in Paraganglia	Associated Neoplasms
Familial PGL 1	SDHD/11q23	Multiple PGL (head and neck)	Thyroid
Familial PGL 2	SDHAF2/11q12.2	Multiple PGL (head and neck)	Unknown
Familial PGL 3	SDHC/1q21-23	Multiple PGL	Unknown
Familial PGL 4	SDHB/1p36	Single PGL	RCC
Familial SDHA-related	SDHA/5p15	Predominant extra-adrenal PGL	GIST
Camey-Stratakis	SDHB, SDHC, SDHD	PGL	GIST
MEN2	RET/2p13-p12	Predominant adrenal Pheo	MTC, parathyroid adenoma, or hyperplasia
VHL	VHL/3p25.3	Predominant adrenal Pheo	Hemangioblastoma, renal cell carcinoma, cysts
NF1	NF1/17q11.2	Predominant adrenal Pheo	Glioma, neurofibromas
Familial KIF1B-related	KIF1B/1p36.2	Predominant adrenal Pheo	Familial KIF1B-related
Familial Pheo 2q	TMEM127/2q11.2	Predominant adrenal Pheo	Unknown
Familial MAX-related	MAX/14q23	Predominant adrenal Pheo	Unknown
Familial PHD2-related	PHD2/1q42.1	Hereditary paraganglioma/pheochromocytoma syndromes	Erythrocytosis

Fig. 12. MEN2: the histopathological features of a MEN2-associated pheochromocytoma are similar to their sporadic counterparts; however, these tumors are usually associated with hyaline globules (H&E, magnification ×400).

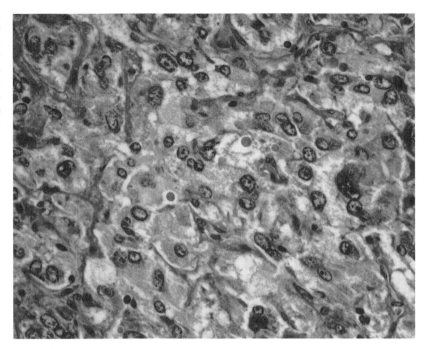

syndromes is largely based on physical examination, family history, imaging, laboratory, and molecular genetic testing. Three types of familial paraganglioma syndromes, (PGL 1, PGL 3, and PGL 4) are recognized with different underlying gene mutations (*SDHD*, *SDHC*, and *SDHB*, respectively).[1,72,73] These genes encode the D, C, and B subunits of succinate dehydrogenase (SDH).

Although patients with all 3 gene mutations can develop pheochromocytomas or paragangliomas within any paraganglion, differences present

Fig. 13. MEN2: cut surface of a pheochromocytoma with areas of degenerative changes and scarring.

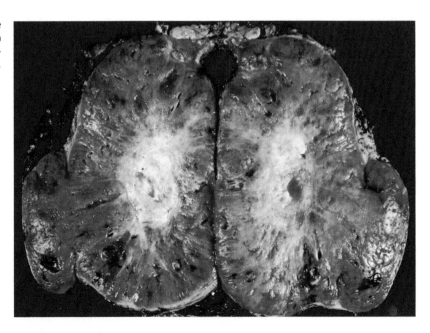

clinically and pathologically with a different gene involved. Mutation in *SDHD* shows parent-of-origin effects. Patients with *SDHB* mutations often present at a young age with multifocal disease and an increased risk of recurrence and malignancy. Patients with *SDHD* and *SDHC* gene mutations often present with head and neck paraganglioma, whereas patients with *SDHB* often present with thoracoabdominal or pelvic paraganglioma. An original study by Dahia and colleagues[72] and other confirmatory findings[73] found that positive immunohistochemistry for SDHB protein (**Fig. 14**) in pheochromocytoma or paraganglioma should lead to *VHL*, *NF1*, and *RET* genetic testing, whereas a negative SDHB stain should lead to *SDH* genetic testing. Early detection through surveillance and removal of tumors may prevent or minimize complications related to mass effects, catecholamine hypersecretion, and malignant transformation.

Other Syndromes

Multiple genes have been implicated in pheochromocytoma and/or paraganglioma in addition to those previously described in syndromes with aberrant expression of *RET*, *VHL*, *NF1*, or the SDH components *SDHA*, *SDHB*, *SDHC*, *SDHD*, and *SDHFA2*. Genetic anomalies more recently identified in association with pheochromocytoma and paraganglioma development include *TMEM127*, *MAX*, *HIF2A*, *KIF1B*, and *PHD2*.

> **Key points**
>
> - Pheochromocytomas and paragangliomas carry the highest degree of heritability in human neoplasms, enabling genetic alterations to be traced to clinical phenotypes.
>
> - Familial pheochromocytomas and paragangliomas comprise more than 30% of all cases.
>
> - Mutations in more than a dozen distinct susceptibility genes have implicated multiple pathways in these tumors, offering insights into kinase downstream signaling interactions and hypoxia regulation.

ENDOCRINE PANCREAS

Pancreatic endocrine tumors originate from the endocrine cells of the pancreas. The cells of origin are located both in the islets and in the epithelium of ducts and ductules. Pancreatic endocrine tumors represent a heterogeneous group of neoplasms showing different morphologic, clinical, and molecular features. Endocrine tumors are subclassified as functioning or nonfunctioning tumors based on the levels of circulating hormone and clinical symptomatology.

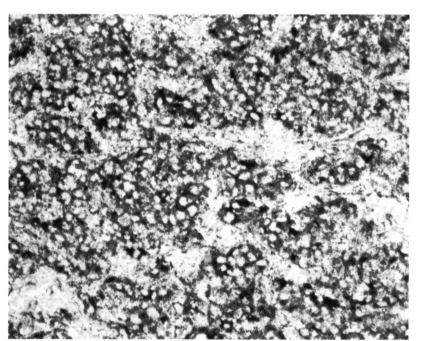

Fig. 14. Paraganglioma in a patient with neurofibromatosis and pheochromocytoma: SDHB by immunostain is retained. Familial syndromes other than those with *SDHx* and some VHL gene mutations show maintained coarse granular immunoreactivity for SDHB (SDHB immunostain, magnification ×100).

Table 10
Pancreatic tumor as part of familial endocrine syndrome

Syndrome	Gene/Chromosomal Location	Pancreatic Pathology
VHL disease	*VHL*/3p25.3	Pancreatic cysts, pancreatic endocrine tumors, presence of clear cells
MEN1	*MEN1*/11q13	Islet-cell hyperplasia, nesidioblastosis, dysplasia; pancreatic endocrine tumors associated with microadenomas
NF1	*NF1*/17q11.2	Somatostatin-producing neuroendocrine tumors
Tuberous sclerosis	*TSC1*/9q34 and *TSC2*/16p13.3	Pancreatic endocrine tumors

ENDOCRINE PANCREATIC TUMOR AS PART OF FAMILIAL ENDOCRINE SYNDROMES

Pancreatic endocrine tumors can occur sporadically or as part of familial disorders (**Table 10**), including MEN1, VHL disease, NF1, and the tuberous sclerosis complex.[74,75] Over the years, increased knowledge in regard to the genetics and molecular pathogenesis of these familial endocrine syndromes provided important insight into the possible pathogenesis of pancreatic endocrine tumor.[1]

Pancreatic Endocrine Tumors in Multiple Endocrine Neoplasia Type 1

Pancreatic involvement in MEN1 patients occurs in 30% to 75% of patients when assessed by clinical screening methods whereas the rate approached 100% in an autopsy series.[76]

Grossly, pancreatic endocrine tumors in MEN1 are usually multiple and variably sized and may be cystic. These tumors clinically can produce different hormones. Histologically, the tumors show a solid, adenomatous, or trabecular pattern. Tumors with amyloid deposition usually exhibit insulin production. A majority of affected patients also exhibit numerous nonfunctioning microadenomas (<0.5 cm) distributed throughout the pancreas, although predominantly in the pancreatic tail. The tumors usually show a distinct trabecular pattern and may show conspicuous connective tissue stroma. In addition to endocrine microadenomas and macrotumors, the pancreas of MEN1 frequently exhibits small nests of endocrine cell budding from ducts and ill-shaped islet-like cell clusters with cellular irregularities and abnormal distribution of the 4 islet cell types.[1,13] Cure is highly dependent on tumor size and early diagnosis in asymptomatic gene carriers.[77]

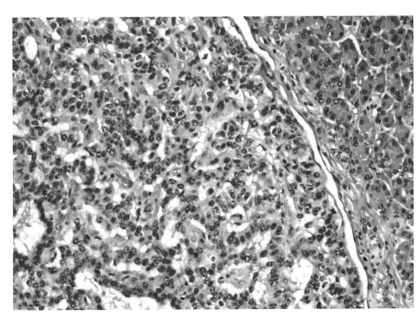

Fig. 15. Pancreas in a patient with VHL disease: marked enlargement of the endocrine islets with maintenance of hormonal cell distribution. This patient had also numerous clear cells and multivacuolated lipid-rich cells (H&E, magnification ×100).

Pancreatic Endocrine Tumors in von Hippel–Lindau Disease

Pancreatic cysts and tumors are both features of VHL disease.[78] Multiple cysts are the most frequent pancreatic manifestation but are rarely of clinical significance and impairment of pancreatic function is uncommon. Pancreatic tumors occur in 5% to 10% of cases, usually non-secretory islet cell tumors.[1] Morphologically, the tumors are typically well circumscribed and often multiple. Tumors are characterized by solid, trabecular, and/or glandular architecture and prominent stromal collagen bands (**Fig. 15**).[1] Immunohistochemically, most tumors are positive for pan-neuroendocrine markers, such as chromogranin A and synaptophysin. By molecular analysis, tumors show allelic loss of the second copy of *VHL*. Pancreatic lesions may precede any other manifestation of VHL disease by several years, and recognition of pancreatic lesions allows earlier diagnosis of VHL.

Other Syndromes

Two other syndromes may be associated with pancreatic endocrine neoplasia: NF1 and tuberous sclerosis (see **Table 10**).

Key points

- In summary, pancreatic endocrine tumors may occur sporadically or as part of familial disorders.

- In familial cases, endocrine tumors are usually multiples and variably sized, may be cystic, and may be associated with islet cell proliferation and microadenomas.

By understanding the pathogenesis of inherited endocrine tumor syndromes and recognizing the unique features of pathologic findings, pathologists have a unique opportunity to provide clinical colleagues guidelines for screening and treatment of the familial endocrine syndromes. There are multiple pathologic findings suggestive of familial endocrine syndromes or for a specific syndrome.

REFERENCES

1. Nosé V, Paner GP, Greenson JK, et al. Diagnostic pathology: familial cancer syndromes. 1st edition. Manitoba (CA): Amirys Publishing, Inc; 2014.
2. Carney JA. Familial multiple endocrine neoplasia: the first 100 years. Am J Surg Pathol 2005;29(2): 254–74.
3. Daly AF, Tichomirowa MA, Beckers A. The epidemiology and genetics of pituitary adenomas. Best Pract Res Clin Endocrinol Metab 2009;23(5):543–54.
4. Burlacu MC, Tichomirowa M, Daly A, et al. Familial pituitary adenomas. Presse Med 2009;38(1):112–6 [in French].
5. Daly AF, Tichomirowa MA, Beckers A. Update on familial pituitary tumors: from multiple endocrine neoplasia type 1 to familial isolated pituitary adenoma. Horm Res 2009;71(Suppl 1):105–11.
6. Daly AF, Beckers A. Update on the treatment of pituitary adenomas: familial and genetic considerations. Acta Clin Belg 2008;63(6):418–24.
7. Verloes A, Stevenaert A, Teh BT, et al. Familial acromegaly: case report and review of the literature. Pituitary 1999;1(3–4):273–7.
8. Dreijerink KM, Varier RA, van Beekum O, et al. The multiple endocrine neoplasia type 1 (MEN1) tumor suppressor regulates peroxisome proliferator-activated receptor gamma-dependent adipocyte differentiation. Mol Cell Biol 2009;29(18):5060–9.
9. Dreijerink KM, Lips CJ, Timmers HT. Multiple endocrine neoplasia type 1: a chromatin writer's block. J Intern Med 2009;266(1):53–9.
10. Dreijerink KM, Hoppener JW, Timmers HM, et al. Mechanisms of disease: multiple endocrine neoplasia type 1-relation to chromatin modifications and transcription regulation. Nat Clin Pract Endocrinol Metab 2006;2(10):562–70.
11. Falchetti A, Marini F, Luzi E, et al. Multiple endocrine neoplasia type 1 (MEN1): not only inherited endocrine tumors. Genet Med 2009;11(12):825–35.
12. Capella C, Riva C, Leutner M, et al. Pituitary lesions in multiple endocrine neoplasia syndrome (MENS) type 1. Pathol Res Pract 1995;191(4):345–7.
13. Nosé V, Erickson LA, Tischler AS, et al. Diagnostic pathology: endocrine. 1st edition. Salt Lake City(UT): Amirsys; 2012.
14. Trouillas J, Labat-Moleur F, Sturm N, et al. Pituitary tumors and hyperplasia in multiple endocrine neoplasia type 1 syndrome (MEN1): a case-control study in a series of 77 patients versus 2509 non-MEN1 patients. Am J Surg Pathol 2008; 32(4):534–43.
15. O'Brien T, O'Riordan DS, Gharib H, et al. Results of treatment of pituitary disease in multiple endocrine neoplasia, type I. Neurosurgery 1996;39(2):273–8 [discussion 278–9].
16. Stratakis CA, Kirschner LS, Carney JA. Clinical and molecular features of the Carney complex: diagnostic criteria and recommendations for patient evaluation. J Clin Endocrinol Metab 2001;86(9):4041–6.
17. Bertherat J. Carney complex (CNC). Orphanet J Rare Dis 2006;1:21.
18. Horvath A, Bossis I, Giatzakis C, et al. Large deletions of the PRKAR1A gene in Carney complex. Clin Cancer Res 2008;14(2):388–95.

19. Stratakis CA, Carney JA, Lin JP, et al. Carney complex, a familial multiple neoplasia and lentiginosis syndrome. Analysis of 11 kindreds and linkage to the short arm of chromosome 2. J Clin Invest 1996;97(3):699–705.
20. Chahal HS, Chapple JP, Frohman LA, et al. Clinical, genetic and molecular characterization of patients with familial isolated pituitary adenomas (FIPA). Trends Endocrinol Metab 2010;21(7):419–27.
21. Tahir A, Chahal HS, Korbonits M. Molecular genetics of the aip gene in familial pituitary tumorigenesis. Prog Brain Res 2010;182:229–53.
22. Tichomirowa MA, Daly AF, Beckers A. Familial pituitary adenomas. J Intern Med 2009;266(1):5–18.
23. Carling T. Molecular pathology of parathyroid tumors. Trends Endocrinol Metab 2001;12(2):53–8.
24. Waldmann J, Lopez CL, Langer P, et al. Surgery for multiple endocrine neoplasia type 1-associated primary hyperparathyroidism. Br J Surg 2010;97(10): 1528–34.
25. Marini F, Falchetti A, Del Monte F, et al. Multiple endocrine neoplasia type 2. Orphanet J Rare Dis 2006;1:45.
26. Santoro M, Melillo RM, Carlomagno F, et al. Molecular biology of the MEN2 gene. J Intern Med 1998; 243(6):505–8.
27. Lakhani VT, You YN, Wells SA. The multiple endocrine neoplasia syndromes. Annu Rev Med 2007; 58:253–65.
28. Bhadada SK, Rao DS. Hyperparathyroidism-jaw tumor syndrome. Endocr Pract 2009;15(3):276–7 [author reply: 277].
29. Iacobone M, Masi G, Barzon L, et al. Hyperparathyroidism-jaw tumor syndrome: a report of three large kindred. Langenbecks Arch Surg 2009;394(5): 817–25.
30. Stalberg P, Carling T. Familial parathyroid tumors: diagnosis and management. World J Surg 2009; 33(11):2234–43.
31. Guarnieri V, Scillitani A, Muscarella LA, et al. Diagnosis of parathyroid tumors in familial isolated hyperparathyroidism with HRPT2 mutation: implications for cancer surveillance. J Clin Endocrinol Metab 2006;91(8):2827–32.
32. Hannan FM, Nesbit MA, Christie PT, et al. Familial isolated primary hyperparathyroidism caused by mutations of the MEN1 gene. Nat Clin Pract Endocrinol Metab 2008;4(1):53–8.
33. Mizusawa N, Uchino S, Iwata T, et al. Genetic analyses in patients with familial isolated hyperparathyroidism and hyperparathyroidism-jaw tumour syndrome. Clin Endocrinol (Oxf) 2006;65(1):9–16.
34. Pollak MR, Chou YH, Marx SJ, et al. Familial hypocalciuric hypercalcemia and neonatal severe hyperparathyroidism. Effects of mutant gene dosage on phenotype. J Clin Invest 1994;93(3): 1108–12.
35. Hendy GN, Guarnieri V, Canaff L. Calcium-sensing receptor and associated diseases. Prog Mol Biol Transl Sci 2009;89:31–95.
36. Hendy GN, D'Souza-Li L, Yang B, et al. Mutations of the calcium-sensing receptor (CASR) in familial hypocalciuric hypercalcemia, neonatal severe hyperparathyroidism, and autosomal dominant hypocalcemia. Hum Mutat 2000;16(4):281–96.
37. Davies L, Welch HG. Increasing incidence of thyroid cancer in the United States, 1973-2002. JAMA 2006;295(18):2164–7.
38. Richards ML. Familial syndromes associated with thyroid cancer in the era of personalized medicine. Thyroid 2010;20(7):707–13.
39. Alsanea O, Clark OH. Familial thyroid cancer. Curr Opin Oncol 2001;13(1):44–51.
40. Alsanea O. Familial nonmedullary thyroid cancer. Curr Treat Options Oncol 2000;1(4):345–51.
41. Dotto J, Nose V. Familial thyroid carcinoma: a diagnostic algorithm. Adv Anat Pathol 2008;15(6): 332–49.
42. Nose V. Thyroid cancer of follicular cell origin in inherited tumor syndromes. Adv Anat Pathol 2010; 17(6):428–36.
43. Nose V. Familial follicular cell tumors: classification and morphological characteristics. Endocr Pathol 2010;21(4):219–26.
44. Jelsig AM, Qvist N, Brusgaard K, et al. Hamartomatous polyposis syndromes: a review. Orphanet J Rare Dis 2014;9(1):101.
45. Harach HR, Soubeyran I, Brown A, et al. Thyroid pathologic findings in patients with Cowden disease. Ann Diagn Pathol 1999;3(6):331–40.
46. Laury AR, Bongiovanni M, Tille JC, et al. Thyroid pathology in PTEN-hamartoma tumor syndrome: characteristic findings of a distinct entity. Thyroid 2011;21(2):135–44.
47. Nose V. Familial non-medullary thyroid carcinoma: an update. Endocr Pathol 2008;19(4):226–40.
48. Zambrano E, Holm I, Glickman J, et al. Abnormal distribution and hyperplasia of thyroid C-cells in PTEN-associated tumor syndromes. Endocr Pathol 2004;15(1):55–64.
49. Harach HR, Lesueur F, Amati P, et al. Histology of familial thyroid tumours linked to a gene mapping to chromosome 19p13.2. J Pathol 1999;189(3): 387–93.
50. Half E, Bercovich D, Rozen P. Familial adenomatous polyposis. Orphanet J Rare Dis 2009;4:22.
51. Groen EJ, Roos A, Muntinghe FL, et al. Extra-intestinal manifestations of familial adenomatous polyposis. Ann Surg Oncol 2008;15(9):2439–50.
52. Harb WJ, Sturgis EM. Differentiated thyroid cancer associated with intestinal polyposis syndromes: a review. Head Neck 2009;31(11):1511–9.
53. Harach HR, Williams GT, Williams ED. Familial adenomatous polyposis associated thyroid

carcinoma: a distinct type of follicular cell neoplasm. Histopathology 1994;25(6):549–61.

54. Stratakis CA, Courcoutsakis NA, Abati A, et al. Thyroid gland abnormalities in patients with the syndrome of spotty skin pigmentation, myxomas, endocrine overactivity, and schwannomas (Carney complex). J Clin Endocrinol Metab 1997;82(7): 2037–43.

55. Kopp P, Pesce L, Solis SJ. Pendred syndrome and iodide transport in the thyroid. Trends Endocrinol Metab 2008;19(7):260–8.

56. Dossena S, Rodighiero S, Vezzoli V, et al. Functional characterization of wild-type and mutated pendrin (SLC26A4), the anion transporter involved in Pendred syndrome. J Mol Endocrinol 2009;43(3):93–103.

57. Ishikawa Y, Sugano H, Matsumoto T, et al. Unusual features of thyroid carcinomas in Japanese patients with Werner syndrome and possible genotype-phenotype relations to cell type and race. Cancer 1999;85(6):1345–52.

58. Charkes ND. On the prevalence of familial nonmedullary thyroid cancer in multiply affected kindreds. Thyroid 2006;16(2):181–6.

59. Bakhsh A, Kirov G, Gregory JW, et al. A new form of familial multi-nodular goitre with progression to differentiated thyroid cancer. Endocr Relat Cancer 2006;13(2):475–83.

60. Uchino S, Noguchi S, Kawamoto H, et al. Familial nonmedullary thyroid carcinoma characterized by multifocality and a high recurrence rate in a large study population. World J Surg 2002;26(8):897–902.

61. Alsanea O, Wada N, Ain K, et al. Is familial nonmedullary thyroid carcinoma more aggressive than sporadic thyroid cancer? A multicenter series. Surgery 2000;128(6):1043–50 [discussion: 1050–41].

62. McKay JD, Lesueur F, Jonard L, et al. Localization of a susceptibility gene for familial nonmedullary thyroid carcinoma to chromosome 2q21. Am J Hum Genet 2001;69(2):440–6.

63. Malchoff CD, Sarfarazi M, Tendler B, et al. Papillary thyroid carcinoma associated with papillary renal neoplasia: genetic linkage analysis of a distinct heritable tumor syndrome. J Clin Endocrinol Metab 2000;85(5):1758–64.

64. Bignell GR, Canzian F, Shayeghi M, et al. Familial nontoxic multinodular thyroid goiter locus maps to chromosome 14q but does not account for familial nonmedullary thyroid cancer. Am J Hum Genet 1997;61(5):1123–30.

65. Pacini F, Castagna MG, Cipri C, et al. Medullary thyroid carcinoma. Clin Oncol (R Coll Radiol) 2010;22(6):475–85.

66. Kloos RT, Eng C, Evans DB, et al. Medullary thyroid cancer: management guidelines of the American Thyroid Association. Thyroid 2009; 19(6):565–612.

67. Libe R, Fratticci A, Bertherat J. Adrenocortical cancer: pathophysiology and clinical management. Endocr Relat Cancer 2007;14(1):13–28.

68. Libe R, Bertherat J. Molecular genetics of adrenocortical tumours, from familial to sporadic diseases. Eur J Endocrinol 2005;153(4):477–87.

69. Haase M, Willenberg HS. Adrenal cortical tumors and multiple endocrine neoplasia-related syndromes. Minerva Endocrinol 2009;34(2):123–35.

70. Choufani S, Shuman C, Weksberg R. Beckwith-Wiedemann syndrome. Am J Med Genet C Semin Med Genet 2010;154C(3):343–54.

71. Karakas Z, Tugcu D, Unuvar A, et al. Li-Fraumeni syndrome in a Turkish family. Pediatr Hematol Oncol 2010;27(4):297–305.

72. Dahia PL, Ross KN, Wright ME, et al. A HIF1alpha regulatory loop links hypoxia and mitochondrial signals in pheochromocytomas. PLoS Genet 2005;1(1):72–80.

73. van Nederveen FH, Gaal J, Favier J, et al. An immunohistochemical procedure to detect patients with paraganglioma and phaeochromocytoma with germline SDHB, SDHC, or SDHD gene mutations: a retrospective and prospective analysis. Lancet Oncol 2009;10(8):764–71.

74. Jensen RT, Berna MJ, Bingham DB, et al. Inherited pancreatic endocrine tumor syndromes: advances in molecular pathogenesis, diagnosis, management, and controversies. Cancer 2008;113(Suppl 7):1807–43.

75. Alexakis N, Connor S, Ghaneh P, et al. Hereditary pancreatic endocrine tumours. Pancreatology 2004;4(5):417–33 [discussion: 434–5].

76. Ekeblad S. Islet cell tumours. Adv Exp Med Biol 2010;654:771–89.

77. Tisell LE, Ahlman H. Treatment of the pancreatic disease of multiple endocrine neoplasia type 1 (MEN 1). Acta Oncol 1989;28(3):415–7.

78. Hough DM, Stephens DH, Johnson CD, et al. Pancreatic lesions in von Hippel-Lindau disease: prevalence, clinical significance, and CT findings. AJR Am J Roentgenol 1994;162(5):1091–4.

Index

Note: Page numbers of article titles are in **boldface** type.

A

Adenoma(s), parathyroid, 518–523.See also
    Parathyroid adenoma.
  pituitary, 577–580
  pituitary, familial isolated, 579–580
Adrenal cortex, 589
  adrenocortical tumor in familial endocrine
    syndromes, 589–591
    in Beckwith-Wiedemann syndrome, 589–590
    in Li-Fraumeni syndrome, 590–591
    primary pigmented nodular adrenocortical
      disease in Carney complex, 590–592
Adrenal medulla paraganglioma, in familial endocrine
  syndromes, 590–594
  hyperplasia and pheochromocytoma in MEN2,
    590–591, 593
Adrenocortical neoplasia, assessing biological
  aggression in, **533–541**
  differential diagnosis of, 533–535
  key features of, 534
Adrenocortical tumors, biological aggression
  assessment of, histology and
  immunohistochemistry in, 537–538
    mitotic grade in, 537, 547
    molecular methods in, 538
    related proliferation-based scoring methods in,
      538
    routine grading of, 538–539
    steroidogenic factor-1 in, 537–538
  malignant potential assessment of, genome-wide
    gene expression profiling studies in, 535–536
    Ki-67 immunohistochemistry in, 535, 537
    molecular methods in, 545–546
    reverse transcription-polymerase chain
      reaction assay in, 536
    routine histology in, 535–536
Anaplastic thyroid carcinoma (ATC), poorly
  differentiated thyroid carcinoma *vs.*, 482–483, 486
  tumor-associated inflammatory cells in, 511
  tumor-associated macrophages in, 506

B

Beckwith-Wiedemann syndrome, 589–590

C

Carney complex, adrenocortical disease in, primary
  pigmented nodular, 590–592

defined, 578, 582, 585–586
  thyroid-associated, 595–596
Chronic lymphocytic thyroiditis, natural killer cells in,
  508
  regulatory cells in, 508
  T lymphocytes in, 507–508

D

Dendritic cells, in normal thyroid gland, 503–506
  in papillary thyroid carcinoma, 503–506
    on CD1a immunostain, 593–594

F

Famiial hypocalciuric hypercalcemia, 581
Familial endocrine syndrome(s), **577–598**
  adrenal cortex, 589–591
  endocrine pancreas, 594–596
  multiple endocrine neoplasia syndromes,
    summary, 578
  nonmedullary thyroid carcinoma, 581–589
  nonthyroidal tumors, 582–586
  paraganglia and adrenal medulla, 590–594
  parathyroid, 580–581
  pituitary, 577–580
    adenomas in, 579–580
  pituitary adenoma, 577–579
  primary hyperparathyroidism, 577–581
  thyroid, 581–589
Familial neuroendocrine syndrome(s), hereditary
  pheochromocytoma-paraglioma syndromes,
  591–594
    neurofibromatosis type 1, 572, 591, 593
      von Hippel-Lindau disease, 572, 591, 594

G

Gastrinomas, 570
Glucagonoma, 570–571

H

Hyperparathyroidism, **515–531**.See also under
  Parathyroid glands.
Hyperparathyroidism, primary, in familial endocrine
  syndromes, 578, 580–581
    familial hypocalciuric hypercalcemiasevere,
      581

http://dx.doi.org/10.1016/S1875-9181(14)00104-4
1875-9181/14/$ – see front matter © 2014 Elsevier Inc. All rights reserved.

United States Postal Service

Statement of Ownership, Management, and Circulation
(All Periodicals Publications Except Requestor Publications)

1. Publication Title
Surgical Pathology Clinics

2. Publication Number
0 2 5 - 4 7 8

3. Filing Date
9/14/14

4. Issue Frequency
Mar, Jun, Sep, Dec

5. Number of Issues Published Annually
4

6. Annual Subscription Price
$200.00

7. Complete Mailing Address of Known Office of Publication (Not printer) (Street, city, county, state, and ZIP+4®)

Elsevier Inc.
360 Park Avenue South
New York, NY 10010-1710

Contact Person
Stephen R. Bushing

Telephone (Include area code)
215-239-3688

8. Complete Mailing Address of Headquarters or General Business Office of Publisher (Not printer)

Elsevier Inc., 360 Park Avenue South, New York, NY 10010-1710

9. Full Names and Complete Mailing Addresses of Publisher, Editor, and Managing Editor (Do not leave blank)

Publisher (Name and complete mailing address)

Linda Belfus, Elsevier, Inc., 1600 John F. Kennedy Blvd. Suite 1800, Philadelphia, PA 19103-2899

Editor (Name and complete mailing address)

Joanne Husovski, Elsevier, Inc., 1600 John F. Kennedy Blvd. Suite 1800, Philadelphia, PA 19103-2899

Managing Editor (Name and complete mailing address)

Adrianne Brigido, Elsevier, Inc., 1600 John F. Kennedy Blvd. Suite 1800, Philadelphia, PA 19103-2899

10. Owner (Do not leave blank. If the publication is owned by a corporation, give the name and address of the corporation immediately followed by the names and addresses of all stockholders owning or holding 1 percent or more of the total amount of stock. If not owned by a corporation, give the names and addresses of the individual owners. If owned by a partnership or other unincorporated firm, give its name and address as well as those of each individual owner. If the publication is published by a nonprofit organization, give its name and address.)

Full Name	Complete Mailing Address
Wholly owned subsidiary of	1600 John F. Kennedy Blvd, Ste. 1800
Reed/Elsevier, US holdings	Philadelphia, PA 19103-2899

11. Known Bondholders, Mortgagees, and Other Security Holders Owning or Holding 1 Percent or More of Total Amount of Bonds, Mortgages, or Other Securities. If none, check box ☐ None

Full Name	Complete Mailing Address
N/A	

12. Tax Status (For completion by nonprofit organizations authorized to mail at nonprofit rates) (Check one)
The purpose, function, and nonprofit status of this organization and the exempt status for federal income tax purposes:
☐ Has Not Changed During Preceding 12 Months
☐ Has Changed During Preceding 12 Months (Publisher must submit explanation of change with this statement)

PS Form 3526, August 2012 (Page 1 of 3 (Instructions Page 3)) PSN 7530-01-000-9931 PRIVACY NOTICE: See our Privacy policy in www.usps.com

---

13. Publication Title
Surgical Pathology Clinics

14. Issue Date for Circulation Data Below
September 2014

15. Extent and Nature of Circulation

		Average No. Copies Each Issue During Preceding 12 Months	No. Copies of Single Issue Published Nearest to Filing Date
a. Total Number of Copies (Net press run)		792	930
b. Paid Circulation (By Mail and Outside the Mail)	(1) Mailed Outside-County Paid Subscriptions Stated on PS Form 3541. (Include paid distribution above nominal rate, advertiser's proof copies, and exchange copies)	473	477
	(2) Mailed In-County Paid Subscriptions Stated on PS Form 3541 (Include paid distribution above nominal rate, advertiser's proof copies, and exchange copies)		
	(3) Paid Distribution Outside the Mails Including Sales Through Dealers and Carriers, Street Vendors, Counter Sales, and Other Paid Distribution Outside USPS®	50	52
	(4) Paid Distribution by Other Classes Mailed Through the USPS (e.g. First-Class Mail®)		
c. Total Paid Distribution (Sum of 15b (1), (2), (3), and (4)) ▶		523	529
d. Free or Nominal Rate Distribution (By Mail and Outside the Mail)	(1) Free or Nominal Rate Outside-County Copies Included on PS Form 3541	13	1
	(2) Free or Nominal Rate In-County Copies Included on PS Form 3541		
	(3) Free or Nominal Rate Copies Mailed at Other Classes Through the USPS (e.g. First-Class Mail)		
	(4) Free or Nominal Rate Distribution Outside the Mail (Carriers or other means)		
e. Total Free or Nominal Rate Distribution (Sum of 15d (1), (2), (3) and (4)) ▶		13	1
f. Total Distribution (Sum of 15c and 15e) ▶		536	530
g. Copies not Distributed (See instructions to publishers #4 (page #3))		256	400
h. Total (Sum of 15f and g) ▶		792	930
i. Percent Paid (15c divided by 15f times 100) ▶		97.57%	99.81%

16. Total circulation includes electronic copies. Report circulation on PS Form 3526-X worksheet.

17. Publication of Statement of Ownership
If the publication is a general publication, publication of this statement is required. Will be printed in the December 2014 issue of this publication.

18. Signature and Title of Editor, Publisher, Business Manager, or Owner

Stephen R. Bushing – Inventory Distribution Coordinator

Date
September 14, 2014

I certify that all information furnished on this form is true and complete. I understand that anyone who furnishes false or misleading information on this form or who omits material or information requested on the form may be subject to criminal sanctions (including fines and imprisonment) and/or civil sanctions (including civil penalties).

PS Form 3526, August 2012 (Page 2 of 3)

Moving?

Make sure your subscription moves with you!

To notify us of your new address, find your **Clinics Account Number** (located on your mailing label above your name), and contact customer service at:

Email: journalscustomerservice-usa@elsevier.com

800-654-2452 (subscribers in the U.S. & Canada)
314-447-8871 (subscribers outside of the U.S. & Canada)

Fax number: 314-447-8029

Elsevier Health Sciences Division
Subscription Customer Service
3251 Riverport Lane
Maryland Heights, MO 63043

*To ensure uninterrupted delivery of your subscription, please notify us at least 4 weeks in advance of move.

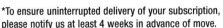

Printed and bound by CPI Group (UK) Ltd, Croydon, CR0 4YY

03/10/2024

01040375-0009